"With grace and humility Elizabeth tells an inspiring story of a mom who set out to intentionally talk with her daughters about sex and sexuality. *Facing "The Talk"* describes what worked and what didn't as Elizabeth sought to negotiate contemporary culture, Christian faith and adolescent sexuality. Above all, Elizabeth shows us a mother who pays attention, who hopes her daughters make different choices than she did and who will love them no matter what choices they make. I highly recommend *Facing "The Talk"* to any mother wanting guidance in the challenge of talking to daughters about sex."
Lisa Graham McMinn, author of *Growing Strong Daughters*

"I've had the privilege of serving students alongside Elizabeth for years. I've watched her heart and insightful wisdom impact countless lives. But the greatest honor I have had is to watch her parent her daughters and to see how they've grown into women who know how to respect and honor their body and sex. I know that I will be using this book in my student ministry and in my home."
Neely McQueen, youth worker, author of *99 Things Every Girl Should Know*

"A few decades ago, there were lots of books helping parents and others to lead their kids through the labyrinth of teenage sexuality. These were, for the most part, self-help books filled with principles and platitudes. As the culture has increasingly pushed against the tried and true messages and strategies of that era, few voices have kept pace. Into this void Elizabeth Chapin brings a fresh, real take on what it means to walk alongside our daughters through today's sexualized and image-defined culture. Using stories and conversations with her own daughters, Chapin's honesty brings hope and reality to what is ultimately more about a journey than a 'talk.' An uplifting correction to the 'add water and stir' bumper stickers of the past, *Facing "The Talk"* helps parents to see up close what it means to be in life with their daughters."
Chap Clark, professor of youth, family and culture, Fuller Theological Seminary, author of *Hurt 2.0: Inside the World of Today's Teenagers*

"Elizabeth Chapin's honest and inviting book demonstrates what it advocates: open, transparent and grace-filled conversations about female embodiment and sex. Chapin's stories of intentional rituals she has practiced with her daughters are grounded in the lavish love of God and told within the context of a loving family and community. She shares her experience, research and counsel with wisdom, humor and humility as she too continues to grow as a daughter of God. A gift well given."
Cherith Fee Nordling, associate professor of theology, Northern Seminary

"Facing "The Talk" is a must-read book for all parents and caregivers of daughters. As a mom, Chapin brings 'The Talk' into the candid arena of everyday life for girls in our hypersexualized, media-drunk culture. Using stories punctuated with the wisdom of her process and the conversation skills she learned helps us to navigate the development of a girl's sexuality together with her faith and family, and not separate from them. Chapin gets extra kudos for not sanitizing the conversation or diminishing the reality that many young girls are sexually exploited by friends and family members."

MaryKate Morse, author, *A Guidebook to Prayer*

"Facing "The Talk" is a book for moms who operate in the real world. This is not a sterile, how-to instructional book, but rather a humorous, candid, insightful look into the mother-daughter relationship as it pertains to discussions of sexuality and sex. Elizabeth Chapin's stories and reflections give me a friend as I face these conversations with my own girls. Her honesty about her own feelings and fumbles in the process forces me to look at my own stuff and to know I'm not alone in the often clumsy world of sex talks."

Alexandra Kuykendall, specialty content editor, MOPS International, author, *The Artist's Daughter*

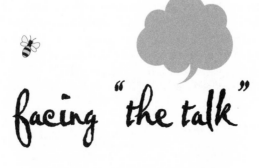

facing "the talk"

CONVERSATIONS WITH MY FOUR DAUGHTERS ABOUT SEX

wendy elizabeth chapin

IVP Books

An imprint of InterVarsity Press
Downers Grove, Illinois

InterVarsity Press
P.O. Box 1400, Downers Grove, IL 60515-1426
ivpress.com
email@ivpress.com

InterVarsity Press® is the book-publishing division of InterVarsity Christian Fellowship/USA®, a movement of students and faculty active on campus at hundreds of universities, colleges and schools of nursing in the United States of America, and a member movement of the International Fellowship of Evangelical Students. For information about local and regional activities, visit intervarsity.org.

All Scripture quotations, unless otherwise indicated, are taken from THE HOLY BIBLE, NEW INTERNATIONAL VERSION®, NIV® Copyright © 1973, 1978, 1984, 2011 by Biblica, Inc.™ Used by permission. All rights reserved worldwide.

While many stories in this book are true, some names and identifying information may have been changed to protect the privacy of individuals.

Cover design: Cindy Kiple
Interior design: Beth McGill

Images: bird and speech bubble: © mxtama/iStockphoto
bumble bees: © lambada/iStockphoto
flying birds: © Jonathan Woodcock/iStockphoto

ISBN 978-0-8308-4322-0 (print)
ISBN 978-0-8308-9910-4 (digital)

Printed in the United States of America ♾

Library of Congress Cataloging-in-Publication Data
Chapin, Wendy Elizabeth, 1964-
  Facing the talk : conversations with my four daughters about sex / Wendy Elizabeth Chapin.
    pages cm
  Includes bibliographical references.
  ISBN 978-0-8308-4322-0 (pbk. : alk. paper)
    1. Sex—Religious aspects—Christianity. 2. Sex instruction for girls—Religious aspects—Christianity.
  3. Mothers and daughters—Religious aspects—Christianity. 4. Girls—Religious life. I. Title.
  BT708.C425 2015
  241'.664—dc23

                                                                        2015027308

P 21 20 19 18 17 16 15 14 13 12 11 10 9 8 7 6 5 4 3 2 1

Y 33 32 31 30 29 28 27 26 25 24 23 22 21 20 19 18 17 16 15

To my four daughters, the Chapin Chicks,

Karen, Katie, Kelly and Kimberly—

Your presence in my life has brought me great

joy and shaped me in more ways than

I ever could have imagined.

And to my husband, Ken—

Your loyalty and kindness have provided the stable

ground for me to do this work.

Contents

Learning to Talk

"What size bra do you wear?"

"Who was your first crush?"

"Can I touch your boobs?"

My hands began to tremble a bit as I scrolled through the anonymous questions posed to my oldest daughter on a social media website.

By the time she was sixteen, Karen had been diagnosed with a hormonal imbalance that caused her to gain quite a bit of weight. The weight gain increased her breast size significantly. For most of her life, Karen's red curls had been the focal point of much of the attention she received from others. But that changed—at least for some—when she matured physically.

For some reason I thought Karen could escape the sexual objectification so common in our society today. I was wrong. And I was not prepared for how she became a sex object in the eyes of her peers. Online, Karen was being bombarded with questions even more explicit than those about her boobs, crushes and bra size. I was shocked.

The trembling in my hands didn't stop and my heart sank

as I kept reading. *How do I respond? Who are these boys posting anonymously? Help!*

My husband and I allow our girls to have online social media accounts as long as they include us in their network of friends.[1] When I notice something that concerns me on these sites, I send them a private message. Some conversations are best conducted out of public view.

After my hands stopped trembling, I sent Karen a message.

ME: Karen, I noticed that link to the website with anonymous questions and am concerned with some of the explicit questions. What do you think about those questions? What are you going to do about it?

KAREN: Mom, I know! It's just some stupid boys.

ME: Let's talk about it sometime.

I stalked that social media site for days. (Yes, I'm one of those parents.) And I was impressed by how my daughter responded to the questions, including the ones about her bra size. She demonstrated wisdom beyond her years. Reading her responses helped calm me. I'm not really sure what all I was afraid of in those moments, but one thing I can tell you for sure—I had a lot of fear. It's only now, as I'm writing this book, that I'm discovering the source of some of my fears and how they influenced my parenting.

Sexual Messages

Today's girls are constantly bombarded with sexual messages—at school, through social media, in movies, songs and advertising, and so on. How are we helping them process these messages? What messages are we sending them about healthy sexuality? At what age should we start talking about sex? How do we protect them in this world of anonymous social media sites, sexting, date rape and Internet sex trafficking? Most importantly, how do we empower them to make wise choices about their bodies and sexual expressions and learn to take care of themselves in a world that can feel very unsafe?

The data is pretty consistent—most girls aren't waiting until marriage to have sex. Many aren't even waiting until adulthood! Unfortunately, too many parents don't explicitly talk about sex. Perhaps we're afraid our kids won't listen. Or we won't know what to say. Maybe we're ashamed of something in our past. Or we're paralyzed by our own brokenness because of something terrible that's happened to us. For some of us, our parents never talked about sex and we made all the right choices, so we expect the same outcome for our own girls. Unfortunately, our silence often does more harm than good.

This book is designed to inspire and encourage you to have conversations about sex with your girls that will prepare them to make healthy, wise and informed choices. This book may also help you face your own fears.

There are many influences that will shape a girl's view of sexuality unless we offer her an alternative—not just an alternative set of rules and regulations, but an alternative imagination, a reframing of the questions about sexuality and a reorienting of sex from what western media culture defines it to be. We need to invite our girls to write their own sexual narrative in light of their participation in a story that is bigger than they are—God's story of creative goodness for the world. But before we can invite them into this bigger story, we have to know our own place in it.

This is not your typical parenting book. I am not an expert sex educator or youth minister. I am a mom. This is my account of how I have developed as a parent and how my development has shaped and formed my ideas about sex. It's about life with four daughters. As my daughters grew and changed, so did I. This book is as much about the process of maturing as a parent as it is about girls maturing into young women.

There are plenty of parenting books on childhood development and I recommend you read a few. But that's not the focus here. This book is a collection of stories. Through reading my stories you may be inspired with ideas for conversations with your own girls, but I do not provide specific content for your conversations. Each family is unique. Your family of origin, marital status, faith tradition and social location, as well as the specific needs and interests of your own girls, will influence what you focus on in your conversations. In appendix A, I offer resources to help you be prepared for the many conversations you will have.

But before we get started with my stories, let me introduce you to the main characters.

About Me

I am the mother of four daughters. My husband, Ken, and I met at work, where I was a technical writer and he was a programmer. We have been married for twenty-two years. We have lived in the Seattle area for more than twenty years and have served at our local church in a variety of ministries. Before I married, I thought I was going to be a missionary to China. God had other plans. Ken serves in our youth ministry, while I serve in our young adult ministry. I am no longer a technical writer; instead I write about faith and culture. I am also an educator, teaching ministry leadership classes online for George Fox Evangelical Seminary and continuing my graduate studies in religion and gender at the University of Washington.

About My Girls

People often talk about our family as a family of redheaded girls. But my daughters don't all have the same kind of red hair—each head of hair is unique. Likewise, my daughters are all unique and amazing young women. I like to refer to us as the Chapin Chicks.

Karen, age twenty-two. When I was a teen, I permed and colored my hair to make it more red and more curly. Only God knew how much I loved curly red hair. Perhaps it was Anne of Green Gables who inspired my love of red hair. Well, Karen has the exact kind of curly red hair I always dreamed of having. She is truly a gift from God. She is studying communication, history and Spanish at Seattle Pacific University. She's an intern at our local church, enjoys hiking and going on adventures with friends, takes amazing photographs, and serves at an orphanage in Mexico on many of her breaks from college. Her favorite Disney character is Merida.

Katie, age twenty. Katie has red curly hair too, but not quite as red or curly as her older sister. It's more like a strawberry blonde, and she prefers to straighten it. Katie was on the gymnastics team in high school and loves to be active. She is studying film at Montana State University in Bozeman. She loves the outdoors and has taken up skiing as a hobby. Among her favorite movies are *The Lord of the Rings* and *The Hobbit*.

Kelly, age eighteen. When Kelly was a baby, her hair was redder and curlier than it is now, but people still see red in it. Kelly is an avid reader and a bright student. Her favorite thing to do is take care of kids. She works part-time at a Montessori preschool and babysits often. She has served in our church nursery since she was a preteen. Her favorite books are based on Greek mythology.

Kimberly, age sixteen. Kimberly is the least curly and the least red of the four redheads. She has red highlights, along with gold and blonde, mixed in with her light brown hair. She looks the most like me when I was young. Kimberly recently sprang up as the tallest of the four girls and is a born leader. She has shown an interest in biology and chemistry and is considering pursuing a career in the medical field. When she's not studying, she likes to spend her time tweeting and watching Patrick Dempsey movies.

I've provided these snapshots of my daughters to remind you that all these stories have a unique context. My hope is that my experiences will inspire you in your unique context. Some challenges we face as parents are similar and many parents share common joys. But I want to avoid the trap of thinking that there's one right way, one best way, one godly path or one "real" way of talking about sex. I don't ever want to presume that I know or understand "God's way" in this matter. God has created humans with infinite variety and calls each of us to be cooperative friends of Jesus, living lives of creative goodness in the power of the Holy Spirit for the sake of others.[2] The uniqueness of each of my daughters is part of God's creative goodness; the ways I interact with them are part of my cooperation with God. I hope my stories will inspire you to create goodness around the topic of sex for the sake of your own daughters.

The stories in this book are not linear—they are topical by age group. By the time I have the first sex talk with my youngest daughter, I've made it through many sex talks with my oldest daughter. You may have heard that a hundred one-minute conversations are better than one hundred-minute conversation about sex, but I suggest that both are necessary. There's something significant that happens to both you and your daughter in the midst of a focused talk about sex. And there's something magical about the moments when conversations about sex just happen in your everyday life. I encourage you to be intentional about both kinds of sex talks.

I'd also like to remind you that often we talk about sex in subtle ways without realizing it. Hopefully my stories will inspire you to capture those magical moments, prepare you for the focused conversations, and help you recognize how and when sex subtly influences the way we talk with our girls.

Intentional Getaways

I took each of my girls on two intentional getaways to talk about sex. But doing something that fits your budget and lifestyle is more important than the time or place. The key is to have intentional, focused conversations. If you're working two jobs just to pay the bills, a few scheduled walks around the block to talk about sex might be the getaway that works best for you. By doing something above and beyond your normal routine, you communicate that these intentional conversations are important. Another approach might be to schedule some extra time on the way to a regular extracurricular activity or church event for a month. Or you could pick one night a month for a few months to have a slumber party in the family room with your girl. Whatever you do, the intentionality and the time together are more important than the location and the activities.

I scheduled the first getaways with my girls prior to their

exposure to sex education in our local school, which in our district takes place in fifth and sixth grade. This first getaway was a time to talk about the birds and the bees. I scheduled the second getaway in early junior high, usually after they started their first period. This second getaway was a time to talk about purity, sexual maturing and temptation. I was preparing to take Karen on her second getaway a few weeks before Katie's first getaway when Katie made a brilliant observation. The three of us were discussing travel plans in the kitchen.

"So, Mom, when we're eleven you tell us how to and when we're thirteen you tell us how *not* to?" Katie asked.

Karen snorted. I laughed a bit nervously. Katie was just entering her snarky phase.

"Yes, Katie, that's right. Maybe we should call them the 'How-To' and the 'How-Not-To' talks instead of 'The Birds and the Bees' and 'The Purity Talk'?"

We all laughed together.

Here's an example of a schedule for getaways:

"The Talk" Part 1: The How-To Sex Talk. Around the age of ten or eleven, but could be scheduled as early as age nine.

"The Talk" Part 2: The How-Not-To Sex Talk. Around the age of thirteen or as a celebration of starting menses.

I have divided the content in the book according to these time points.

Throughout the text I will include the following hashtags to highlight important concepts. For the purposes of the book these callouts are longer than tweets, but please do follow me on Twitter, @facingthetalk.

#facingthetalk includes advice on important things to consider or do along with what you might want to rethink or avoid.

#selfcare includes suggestions on how and when you might want to create time and space for adequate self care.

Talking Topics

In appendix C you'll find a list of topics I recommend parents think about. Some will be covered in more detail in this book; others are merely mentioned. You don't need to talk about every topic on the list. Some may not even seem explicitly related to sex. When this explicit connection is not clear, I'll attempt to explain how and why I think the topic is relevant. You may want to talk about other topics that aren't covered in this book. I encourage you to seek out a variety of resources to inform and equip you in this important parenting task.

This is a book about sex. Sexual content is found on every page. I will be honest and open about my personal sexual past as well as straightforward about what's going on with my daughters. I have talked with them and my husband about the stories I'm including in this book and they have given their consent to their telling. Each story shared is designed to help make a point more clearly. This may feel disconcerting at times, especially if you live in an environment where talking about sex is taboo. I encourage you to pay attention to how you feel when reading the stories, especially those you react to strongly. Your reaction is a good indication of topics you may need to think about more deeply or personal boundaries you may need to set.

If you're unfamiliar with the concept of boundaries, I encourage you to seek out resources that will help you learn more—there are many available.[3] It's important for parents to understand the idea of boundaries, especially when they're talking about sex. Some parents view their children as extensions of themselves. They control their children through fear and shame, tell them they're making the parent angry, and often teach them to be responsible for the parent's feelings instead of their own. A lack of personal boundaries often indicates en-meshment and codependency.[4] It's difficult to teach our children to have healthy sexual boundaries if we do not first teach them to have healthy personal boundaries. They need to know who and what they are responsible for.

When we talk with our girls about sex, our thinking is influ-enced by our own past experiences, and we need to be honest with ourselves about how this affects our interactions with our daughters. Sometimes this means unearthing painful memories. Other times it means opening our eyes to realities that didn't exist when we were their age. Often it means letting go of some ideal sexual story we imagine for our girls. I encourage you to create time and space for adequate self care as issues from your own past surface.

I witnessed my sister being sexually molested when I was eight and she was eleven. That traumatic experience has had a lasting effect on both of us. One in four girls is sexually abused by the time she is eighteen years old. Nearly one in five women has been raped sometime in her life, and most victims of rape or sexual assault are women under the age of twenty-four. I separate these statistics because rape and sexual abuse are similar, yet different. Rape is a form of sexual abuse, but other types of unwanted sexual contact are abuse as well. My sister was not raped. My father touched her inappropri-ately. And it happened to her repeatedly between the ages of nine and eleven.

It's important to talk about this distinction so our girls can recognize the signs of sexual abuse early. It's also important to help them understand that rape is not always violent in the sense of being forced to have sex at gunpoint or knifepoint. Date rape and consensual sexual activity between a minor and an adult are types of rape in which overt force or threat may not be present. We need to talk to our daughters about abuse at age-appropriate times. But it's never too early to begin to talk with them about consent.

We also need to talk with our daughters about domestic violence. My father was physically violent with my mother and emotionally controlling. I witnessed these things as a young girl, and I wish someone had talked to me about abuse then. You may have gone through a similar experience, and you may encounter material in this text that triggers trauma from your own past. I encourage you to talk to a safe person who can help you process these emotions as they occur. Abuse and trauma tend to be repeated and reenacted in various ways, and we must be aware of their staying power and work to break their destructive force in our lives.

Unfortunately the feelings of fear and shame that I experienced are common. You may not have experienced trauma or abuse in your past, but you may have some fear or shame that keeps you from talking with your daughter about sex. Hopefully my stories of how I faced my fear and shame will help you face yours.

Many parents fear their daughters will engage in risky sexual behaviors. This fear is not unfounded. Taking sexual risks can result in unintended health problems, sexually transmitted disease and unwanted pregnancy. And many factors are out of a parent's or adolescent's control. For example, early maturation may be connected with earlier sexual activity. Age of maturation is controlled by genetics, not by choice. Peer influence and drug and alcohol use are also linked with earlier sexual activity. Parents can attempt to control these factors, but ultimately those are choices our children will make themselves. Fortunately, some factors are under parental control. For example, parental supervision and social bonds with religious and family institutions are connected with later sexual behavior.[5] We can choose to supervise our children and engage in activities that promote family bonding.

Because I was a victim of trauma and abuse, it was easy for me to fear things that were out of my control. In fact, it's common for people to respond to abuse by trying to control things in their environment. Unfortunately, such controlling responses do not promote health and healing and often serve to perpetuate abusive systems. You may have heard it said that worry is taking responsibility for things you have no control over. It may seem obvious to say this, but it's true: We cannot control everything. Nor are we expected to. While the platitude "God is in control" is not always helpful, I do find it comforting to know that God is with me, helping me to know what things are my responsibility and what things are not.

The pressures of married life with small children brought up many tensions that eventually led me to seek help through counseling. Even those who have not experienced trauma and abuse as children deal with the tension of the differences between their own upbringing and their context as parents. For some the tension is intense enough to require professional help. In raising children, we need all the help we can get. I hope this book helps you as a parent recognize those times when you might need to seek support from others.

Sex is a complicated topic. In many church contexts it's considered taboo, but it's everywhere in the mainstream media. Even in our own lives sex is confusing at times. Is it what we do or who we are? Who defines sex—the church, the society we live in, our family? What does it mean to have sex? Here are some terms that will help orient you as you begin this journey with me through the stories of my sex talks with my girls.

Defining Sex and Sexuality

Sex and sexuality include:

- Being male or female—differences and similarities
- Body image
- Relationships with others
- How we grow and change over the years
- How we reproduce
- Personality, communication, expression, values
- Our embodied interaction with the world around us

Here are some other concepts to keep in mind:

- Biological sex refers to sex organs and other physical factors. Biological sex is determined by genetics and development before birth.

- Gender roles involve the characteristics a culture connects with masculinity or femininity. Gender roles are primarily socially constructed and vary across time and place.

- Gender identity refers to a private sense of maleness or femaleness that may or may not match biological sex.

- Sexual identity refers to sexual orientation or the orientation of attraction and sexual desire.

- Gender and sexual identities are influenced by biological, psychological and sociological factors.

Often when we use the term "sex" in everyday language, we are talking about sexual intercourse. And by sexual intercourse, we are referring to a penis-inserted-into-a-vagina kind of sexual intercourse. However, talking about sex is much more complicated than talking about sexual intercourse. When I first started discussing sex with my oldest daughter, we mostly talked about sexual intercourse. Over the years these talks have come to encompass much more. I have learned a lot over the years, and I hope that you, like me, will grow and learn alongside your daughter as you talk with her about sex.

Throughout this book I will refer to mothers, fathers and daughters. I recognize that half of the population exists in nontraditional family situations. But I will use these terms for the sake of simplicity, trusting that you will adapt them to your unique situation. For those in blended families, the relationships between stepparents and biological parents can be complicated. Adoptive parents have another set of challenges. Single parents might find it helpful to invite a good friend to join in conversations with their girl about sex. You'll also notice that I often use the word "girl" instead of "daughter." This is intentional. Some of you are foster parents or hope to be a resource for a niece or granddaughter. Others may want to help a girl in their small group from church. Whatever your role, I hope you will find encouragement in these pages.

An Invitation

I invite you to join me on this complex and often scary journey of talking to girls about sex. As we explore new territory, revisit our own stories and encounter new paths along the way, may we do so with grace, hope, love and faith. I pray you will open your heart to God's healing and liberating power and be inspired to imagine new kingdom realities. Cultivating a new kingdom imagination doesn't happen overnight and it doesn't happen without wrestling with complexity and diversity in an ever-changing world.

Remember, when we're helping our girls process the sexual messages they encounter on a regular basis, intentional longer conversations are as important as the magical moments that occur throughout the day. Considering what we say and how we say it is crucial. It may seem at times that we live in a world of impossible sexual choices. When we begin to feel anxious, may we never forget that with God all things are possible—including talking with girls about sex.

The How-To Sex Talk

y personal history played a big part in my decision to
take Karen on an intentional getaway to talk about sex.
But it was not the only influence. In my women's Bible study
groups, I had already heard some of my friends debating
whether to allow their children to attend sex ed classes at
school. I had friends on all sides of the issue, but the majority
of them homeschooled, sent their kids to private Christian
school, or signed a waiver to keep their child out of public
school sex ed classes. I understood and respected their decisions, but Ken and I had our own decision to make.

We have always believed that it was our responsibility as
parents to educate our children, whether about religion and
spirituality, math and science, history and language, or sex and
health. We took responsibility for choosing the appropriate
education providers and were engaged parents in both public
school and Sunday school. Some of my friends were concerned
that the public school sex ed curriculum would expose their
kids to information that opposed their beliefs and could potentially cause harm. But I wondered what could be so dangerous

about the public school curriculum.

Ken and I ultimately decided we would do a little bit of both—I would take them on a special getaway to talk about God's plan for sex and then we would let them go through sex ed at school. Our hope was to open up the dialogue with our daughters so that if they were exposed to ideas that conflicted with our beliefs, we would be able to talk about it.

How-To Sex Talk No. 1

At the end of our first cross-country family vacation, I planned a road trip with my firstborn daughter, who was then ten years old, to visit my best friend, Tara, in Tennessee by way of Atlanta. While the rest of the family flew home to Seattle from Boston, Karen and I flew to Atlanta.

We spent two days in Atlanta visiting my dad. It had been a few years since Karen had seen her grandpa. He had been diagnosed with Alzheimer's and was no longer able to travel. I wasn't ready to take the younger kids to see him, but Karen was old enough and knew him best.

My sister, Lori, joined us in Atlanta for the weekend. She made the long cross-country trip to be with us because she didn't want to visit our dad alone. Even though she had gone through counseling and reconciled with our father, she still had trouble being alone with him. We had lived in fear for many years.

I'm not sure if Karen was picking up on our anxiety, worried about visiting her sick grandpa or nervous about having the sex talk, but she went sleepwalking during the night after we'd visited my dad. The three of us were sharing a hotel room, and Lori and I awoke when we heard the door catch on the metal bar latch we had secured. Locking our bedroom door was something Lori and I never forgot to do. It was a habit we'd developed after our father molested her.

Lori woke up first. She had always been the one to wake up first. When we were young, our parents would sometimes fight after we went to bed. Lori would comfort me back to sleep before I was even fully awake.

> **#facingthetalk:** Examine your feelings about having the sex talk. Are you anxious about it? Looking forward to it? Avoiding it like the plague? Meticulously planning it years in advance? Some parents avoid the topic out of fear or shame. But fear and shame perpetuate fear and shame. Think about the experiences that have shaped your thinking about sex and pay attention to places you may need healing or help working through your own emotions. Abuse cycles repeat. Trauma is most often passed down from generation to generation. Do what you must to break the cycle.
>
> **#selfcare:** If you have had painful or difficult experiences with sex, be sure to seek help and healing through counseling before you attempt an intentional getaway.

The next day the sun was shining when we arrived at the amusement park, but dark gray clouds were on the horizon. The humidity was so thick it felt like we were slogging through mashed potatoes just to get from one ride to another. We knew those clouds were going to break any minute. I had planned this amusement park visit because I'd read that when you plan an intentional getaway to talk about something nobody wants to talk about, you'd better include something really fun in the trip!

The Dahlonega Mine Train, my childhood favorite, was our first ride. Then we walked as fast as we could to make sure we hit all the roller coasters and thrill rides before we left. We saved the best for last as we were making our way out of the park—the

Acrophobia Ride. Yep, you guessed it—this was a "face your fears" kind of ride. It was a twenty-story tower that took you to the top, then let you freefall straight back down—all while standing up. We were prepared to face our fears when the clouds burst. We arrived at the ride only to find it closed because of the risk of lightning. That was one fear I wasn't ready to face.

"Mom, do we have to leave?" Karen asked. "I really want to do the freefall ride!"

We calculated how long it would take to drive to the airport while we sought shelter from the storm.

I wanted to stay too and experience the thrill of escaping from a tower of fear. But there was no way to know when the threat of lightning would pass.

"I know! I really want to do the freefall ride too," I replied. "I can't believe they just closed the ride. But we don't really have a choice. We have to get Lori to the airport in time to catch her plane. And it's time for us to hit the road to visit Tara in Tennessee."

When I think back to that first intentional mother-daughter getaway to talk about sex, I recognize that firstborns bear the brunt of our trial-and-error parenting, experiencing more trials and errors than their younger siblings as we figure things out. My first error: thinking she would talk to me just because we were trapped in the car on a long road trip. Her first trial: listening to me talk about sex without any opportunity for escape.

But there we were on the road.

"Mom, I don't want to talk about this."

"Well, you don't have to talk if you don't want to. You can just listen." I adjusted the air conditioning vent so it wouldn't blow directly in my face.

I took a deep breath and shot up one of those arrow prayers to God.

Where do I start? What was I thinking when I planned this road trip?

Oh, I remember. I wanted to tell her about God's good intentions for sex before she learned about how the sperm meets the egg in sex ed at school.

Now what was that truth again?

The words came out awkwardly. I said something about God creating sex and sex being good. It's hard to remember the words I actually used—that part is a blur. I was nervous and I hadn't rehearsed a thing!

One thing I do remember: I told her that sex is enjoyable and nothing to be ashamed of.

"Mom, I really don't want to talk about this." Karen put her bare feet on the dash, which was strictly forbidden in the family car.

Instead of asking her to put her filthy feet down, I kept going with my explanation about how sacred and special sex is.

I rambled nervously for what seemed like miles. I hoped she might be ready to talk for a bit.

"I want you to know that you can talk to me about this anytime. Whenever you have questions, you can always ask me. So, do you have any questions?"

I kept my mouth shut as we crossed the border into Tennessee. We still had many miles to go and I feared it was going to be an awkwardly silent ride. By then I was at a loss for words.

I was ready to take the next exit off I-75 to stop for a snack or take a potty break—anything to escape the voiceless tension that filled the car—when Karen broke her vow of silence.

"So, do you and Dad talk?"

I had been imagining questions about penises and vaginas or how the sperm and egg stayed together, but Karen's mind went somewhere else entirely. Her personal and intimate question threw me for a loop. She wasn't concerned with mechanics; she wanted to know about love.

"Um, uh, well, yes, we talk. I mean, not the whole time, but we talk to each other while having sex."

One of the purposes of this first sex talk is to open up the conversation and remove the taboo from the topic. I have always been forthright in answering my girls' questions in age-appropriate ways as they come up, but this conversation felt extra important. I fumbled through a disjointed explanation of the beauty of the human body and how amazingly it works and how sex is not just about making babies or bodily pleasure but an expression of love and intimacy.

This first sex talk is probably not the time to go into intimate details about the range of behaviors possible in the bedroom and what kind of expectations are appropriate. It is, however, the right time to locate sex in the context of relationship. Sex is a physical act, but it is never *just* a physical act. It is a relational act with significant physical components.

Relationships and bonding are integral to what it means to be human. We are more than our bodies and our instincts. Our girls hear many messages in their formative years indicating that sexual intercourse is a natural thing and even necessary for them to be healthy and happy. They might hear from their friends or media sources that if they're deprived of sex or deprive themselves of it, something is wrong with them. They might hear that having sex is a normal part of adolescent behavior and is kind of like exercising—that's something one of my own daughters heard when she was in fifth grade!

One thing I hoped to do for my girls was to identify sexual intercourse as a healthy and joyful part of an intimate, com-

mitted love relationship, but not an essential part. Sexual intercourse certainly facilitates bonding and intimacy, but there are
many other ways to bond through loving touches, both sexual
and nonsexual. Strong emotional bonds between parents and
children help children grow up with the capacity to bond non-
sexually with others. And one of the main purposes of these
intentional getaways is to facilitate bonding with your daughter.

> **#facingthetalk:** A fun, relaxing, safe and mutually enjoyable context
> can create space for fruitful conversation. Include activities that promote
> bonding. Your getaway is not just about talking. Laughing, hugging,
> singing silly songs, watching a sunset together and many other activi-
> ties encourage bonding and connection as well. Resist the temptation
> to focus on the content while ignoring the context.

Reflection. Looking back, I wonder if I should have done this
first sex talk a year earlier when Karen was not so oppositional.
The differences between a nine-year-old and a ten-year-old are
pretty significant. Nine-year-olds still define themselves by who
they're similar to and who they're connected to; ten-year-olds
are beginning to define themselves in terms of who they are not.
They don't throw away everything they have assimilated from
their parents, but they don't want to hear it anymore. They want
to start thinking their own thoughts and coming up with their
own ideas. This often manifests in the "I don't want to talk about
it" attitude—an attitude that's especially prevalent in conversations initiated by parents.

   Ten-year-olds also assert their differences and realize their in-
dividuality by saying in subconscious but not always subtle ways,
"I am not like my parents!" Which then morphs into, "I do not like
my parents!" And occasionally into, "I hate you!" Fortunately,
this opposition doesn't last forever—it is a transitional phase into

differentiated mature adulthood. Parenting educator Debra Haffner notes that most teenagers go through a period of seeming to reject the ideas and values of their parents, yet almost all of them adopt very similar values by the time they reach adulthood.[1]

In some ways it was easier to talk about anatomy with Karen, but that's not what she wanted to hear. She wanted to know more about the relational details. Perhaps if we respond to our girls' opposition by inviting them to ask questions, we can enter into a cooperative discussion that contributes to their developing sense of self.

> **#facingthetalk:** Plan ahead and think about what details you feel comfortable sharing about your relationship with your spouse. Talk with your spouse about why sex is important in your relationship. Imagine how you can communicate the love you experience and express through sexual activities with your partner. Remember to explain that the experiences of various couples are different. Your experiences are not a standard but can be an example of a loving sexual relationship. If you're a single parent, talk about how it once was or how you wished it would be. Remember, sex is more than just mechanical details. If you had painful or difficult experiences, be careful not to pass on shame or blame.

How-To Sex Talk No. 2

At least I had a plan this time. I had found a lovely book to read with my daughter Katie, age eleven, on our getaway. It was the third book in the Learning About Sex for Girls series, *How You Are Changing*.[2] It looked good to me. But Katie had other ideas.

"Do we have to read this stupid book? It looks so fake."

Katie had picked the bed closest to the bathroom in our hotel room and lay on her stomach staring at the cover. They say you can't judge a book by its cover, but that didn't stop her from trying.

I plopped down on the bed next to her and offered to read it aloud, like when she was little. I tried to tickle her a bit, but she just grumbled and wiggled away, grabbing the book in a huff.

"Fine. I'll read the first chapter. But then we're going swimming."

Katie buried her head in the book. After a long enough time for me to believe that she'd read it but a short enough time for me to suspect she was just placating me, her head emerged from the pages.

"I told you it was stupid."

She closed the book, grabbed her swimsuit and locked herself in the bathroom to change.

Soon she emerged in her brand-new yellow and blue bikini. I squeezed my body into my one-piece bathing suit with a skirt, the kind that covered my childbirth-widened hips and hid my stretch marks. We grabbed the plush robes and wrapped our bodies in their comfort as we headed to the pool.

We hung our robes on some hooks and waded into the warm mineral waters of the Harrison Hot Springs Resort.

"Do you remember ever seeing your dad naked?" I asked as I glided through the water toward the deep end.

I was curious how much Katie knew about the differences between girls and boys, between women and men. I had experienced a "let's all go skinny-dipping with our parents" kind of adolescence. But that's not what we did around our house. I knew she had seen her dad naked at some point when she was little. We had talked about it back then. But I wondered what she remembered and what she thought about it now.

"Yeah, I remember seeing him naked when I was little. It was no big deal."

She dove under the water and swam around me, taunting me to race her to the waterfall at the other end of the pool. We reached the waterfall and sat listening to it splash around us while the mist floated up above our heads. The chill in the air was as refreshing as the warm mineral waters were rejuvenating. Katie laughed out loud as a memory bubbled up in her like the waters hitting the pool from the waterfall.

"Did I ever tell you about the time our neighbor John showed me his?"

"No!" I waited for her to offer more details, but she glided under the water like a fish.

When she emerged, I asked, "Did you show him yours?"

"No way!" She disappeared under the water again and emerged grabbing my shoulders to try to dunk me.

"Why not?" I started to slip and barely kept my head above water.

She gave up trying to dunk me and swam around me to rest on a ledge. "What did I have to show? It's not like I can whip it out and show it off like he did! Anyway, he'd probably already seen his mom naked and was more interested in showing his than seeing mine."

Reflection. When it comes to body parts, I've always had a hard time using the words "vagina" and "vulva." It seems like male body parts are much more recognizable since they're external. Penis and testicles. You can grab them. But female sex organs seem more complex. The vulva includes the labia, the vagina and the clitoris all in close proximity to the urethra. And then we have uterus and ovaries, fallopian tubes and cervix. I'm sure I am forgetting something. That's why I brought the book with me. That's why I wanted Katie to read the book, even though she thought it was stupid.

One thing I've learned is that these getaways are good times to practice sharing control and giving consent. As the parent I still established the boundaries, but sharing control gave my daughters the opportunity to practice decision making. By asking, "Would you like to read the chapter silently or would you like me to read it aloud to you?" I established the boundary—we *are* reading the book. But I also invited Katie to participate in the process by choosing how she would comply. She was able to consent to reading the book with me on her own terms within the established boundaries. Sharing control is a concept I learned from Love and Logic Parenting, a class and a book that I relied on to learn about parenting.[3]

As with Karen, I wish I had done Katie's getaway a year earlier. But I'd started scheduling these mother-daughter getaways around my girls' birthdays. I had just finished the first How-Not-To talk with Karen a few weeks before at the same resort. Scheduling around birthdays was one way I justified spending the money on an adventure. Again, even if you don't have time or money for a road trip or a weekend getaway at a resort, you can still make the intentional talks special. A trip to the local zoo or a picnic lunch and afternoon hike might be enough to create a significant bond and give you the one-on-one time needed to explore the materials you choose to cover and create space for random conversations to bubble up.

Conversations about body parts often surface around this age, whether you're on a getaway or in the midst of life at home. While it's important to know and name the body parts according to their given names, it's also appropriate to use nicknames. Terms of endearment for sex organs and sexual features is a common practice and not harmful unless the nicknames are derogatory.

Some sex education experts advocate using anatomical terms from even the earliest age. They argue that using other terms cloaks the external genitalia in shame. But my view is that nicknames don't convey shame in every instance. How often do we speak of our baby's cute little tummy or precious toesies? As long as nicknames are used along with anatomical terms, shame will not necessarily follow. But if you find yourself using nicknames because of shame, those issues should be addressed. While we keep our genitals covered with clothes, we need to be careful not to clothe them in shame by refusing to talk about them.

> **#facingthetalk:** Practice using anatomical terms for sexual body parts. Nicknames are fine, but connect them with anatomical terms. Practice using the words "penis" and "vulva" before the getaway. If you have silly or special terms of endearment for external genitalia, connect them explicitly with the anatomical terms. Silence often unintentionally communicates shame and perpetuates fear of the unknown.
>
> **#selfcare:** If you experience intense discomfort talking about body parts, discuss it with a close friend or counselor. When you practice using anatomical terms before the getaway, pay attention to how your body feels. Do you tense up? Do you blush? Do you feel anger or shame? Allow your body to lead you into places where you may need healing and help.

How-To Sex Talk No. 3

Kelly's arrival in our family was unique in a number of ways and marked a turning point in our family system. Once she arrived, my husband and I were outnumbered. We went from feeling like we could manage family life to feeling overwhelmed within months of her birth. And that overwhelmed feeling lasted for years.

While her arrival marked a turning point, it also happened on a very special day—my birthday.

We scheduled our first sex talk getaway right after Kelly's eleventh birthday.

We arrived at Dinah's Garden Hotel and checked into our poolside room. Kelly immediately changed into her bathing suit.

I placed the *How You Are Changing* book on the perfectly made bed.

"Kelly, I'm going to go explore the gardens while you read the first chapter."

She draped herself across the end of the bed and began reading without a peep of resistance. I let out a sigh of relief as I stepped out onto the patio and shut the sliding glass door behind me.

I wandered the gardens, basking in the manicured tranquility. A hummingbird was hovering over an Asiatic lily and all seemed right with the world. I returned to the room hoping Kelly had finished. I was ready to put on my bathing suit and take a swim.

"Mom, did you want to have four girls?" Kelly looked up at me with her bright blue eyes.

The tranquility of the gardens faded as memories of Kelly's early childhood clouded my mind like an approaching storm.

Reflection. Looking back, I realize that fear played a big part in each of my experiences with my daughters, albeit in different ways. With Kelly, my fears kept me waiting as long as possible to have this first sex talk. I had realized that an earlier age would have been better with my older daughters, but I didn't feel that way about Kelly. At age ten, Kelly was still sucking her thumb. What's more, I was afraid that it was my fault. I worried that she struggled with immaturity and insecurity because of something I had done when she was little. Something I had a hard time forgiving myself for. And this fear was why I waited as long as possible to go on our getaway.

As a young adult, I was taught by mentors and Christian counselors that my early sexual experiences were a result of my troubled family relationships. Without knowing other aspects of my life, many Christian leaders who influenced my young adult spiritual development attributed my adolescent sexual promiscuity to factors related to my parents' divorce and the absence of my father during most of my formative years. This lack of connection with my dad, they said, led me to early sexual activity.

This belief persisted in my mind as I parented and increased my fear level significantly. I worried not just about whether my girls felt loved by their dad, but also whether they felt loved by me. This fear at times frustrated me to the point of anger at myself that spilled over onto those closest to me. I often felt like a failure in how I expressed love to my family, especially Kelly. These feelings of failure intensified my fear. I worried that if Kelly felt a lack of love in any way, it would make her vulnerable. She might go looking for love in all the wrong places as I had, or she might accept love from all the wrong places because my love wasn't good enough.

When Kelly asked whether we'd wanted to have four girls, it felt like she was asking, "Mom, did you want *me*?" And the answer to that question was difficult to formulate.

My husband and I practiced natural family planning, trusting God with the timing of our babies. We got pregnant with Kelly just ten months after Katie was born. When we found out, I was upset—I didn't want to have another baby so soon. I wasn't even sure I wanted to have another baby at all. I was overwhelmed with two; how could I handle three? These thoughts led to struggles with fear and shame.

How much of this truth did I need to tell Kelly?

At Dinah's Garden Hotel, I knew I needed to tell her enough of the truth to help her understand. While there were times when she was little that I did things that may have made her feel unwanted, deep down I have always loved and wanted her.

• • •

"Kelly, it's complicated," I said as I sat down next to her on the bed looking out at the pool, trying to recover a bit of that tranquility I'd discovered in the gardens. "Your dad and I didn't really have a plan for how many children we wanted to have. We wanted as many children as God wanted to bless us with. We didn't think much about whether we wanted boys or girls; we knew God would give us whatever was best."

I stroked her long, wavy hair as I tried to explain the complicated thoughts and emotions in my heart.

"Are you ready to go swimming?" I asked. "We can talk more about this later. I know you want to get in that pool."

Kelly rolled off the bed, opened the sliding glass door and bounded across the patio, heading straight for the pool. She splashed into the water and turned around beckoning me to join her. I hesitated at the pool's edge, not quite sure I was ready to join her. I needed to soak in some California sun before I took the plunge.

After swimming for a while, we went to Outback Steakhouse for dinner, ordering a Victoria's Filet with steamed broccoli smothered in butter.

"What do you think about the reading so far?" I asked. Our server had just delivered a loaf of that dark, sweet Bushman bread Outback serves before the main course.

"It's okay. Except the stories are kind of fake. And I already know that God is the one who makes babies. Do we really have to talk about this? Why can't I just learn about it in school?"

"Well, your dad and I want to be the first ones to tell you about important things. That's why your dad taught Sunday school when you were a toddler. He wanted to be the first one to tell you all those Bible stories. We believe that God created sex as a good thing and it's really important to learn about it from God's perspective. So, I wanted to be the first one to talk to you about how your body is changing and how these changes are related to God's plan for sex." I buttered the last piece of bread and took a bite.

"Karen and Katie already told me some stuff and I read Katie's American Girl book."

"Well, the American Girl *Care and Keeping of You* book is a great resource for learning about hygiene, budding breasts and other early physical changes. So where are you on the budding breast scale?"

"Mom, I don't really want to talk about that here! But can we go shopping for a bra? I think I'm in stage two." She blushed as the server arrived with our food.

I waited until the server left to answer her question.

"I bet Katie has grown out of some of her training bras. We could check with her when we get home." Kelly rolled her eyes.

"I don't want hand-me-down bras. I already wear hand-me-down bathing suits. Can we get at least one new bra for me?"

"Okay, we'll look in the mall before we go to the movie. After all, we're celebrating our birthdays. You know I don't really like malls and shopping for clothes, but we can do a little shopping while we're here."

Reflection. One of the important things I began to realize as my girls matured was that their schedule was not always my schedule. I was tempted to make sure we covered every topic I thought was important. But is that even possible? I scheduled the intentional getaways as a bonding experience and an opportunity to expose them to topics that would likely emerge in the coming years. I hoped that the bonding experience of the getaway would foster open communication for those hundreds of one-minute conversations at home.

Books and school curriculums expose our girls to many of the facts. Our conversations help give context to the facts. For example, I hadn't thought to buy Kelly a training bra. I hadn't noticed any budding! As the third daughter, she was exposed to some of the facts earlier than her older sisters might have been, while at the same time blooming a little later. Kelly may not have been interested in talking about the things I thought were important, but there were things she was interested in. And one thing she was interested in was shopping for bras.

When the girls were little, I would meet my friends at the mall and shop for cute girl clothes. I really tried to do what the other moms were doing. But I always felt drained and grumpy after a shopping trip. By the time Kelly was ten, I had discovered that the "women love shopping" stereotype did not apply to me. But Kelly loved fashion and dressing well. She always wore matching outfits and dressed before coming down for breakfast. I knew this was an important opportunity for me to bond with her over something she was interested in.

> **#facingthetalk:** Think about the most important topics you want to discuss with your girl, but be flexible. Disinterest is not a sign of trouble or delayed development. We all develop at different rates—physically, emotionally, intellectually and spiritually. As an adult I am still developing in many ways. And we all have different interests, different things that are important to us. Be open and respectful of your daughter's differences and pay attention to the topics that seem most important to her.

The morning after our dinner, shopping and movie date, I woke Kelly up and asked her to join me for breakfast. Kelly is not a morning person (neither am I), but it was already past ten. We still had things to talk about and one last swim to enjoy before we checked out of the hotel. I walked across the patio to the poolside café and ordered some much-needed coffee.

Fifteen minutes later she joined me. I had already ordered her breakfast, one of her favorites—hash browns smothered in melted cheese.

As soon as her favorite food arrived, Kelly's I'm-not-a-morning-person grumpiness abated.

"Has the book gotten any better? Do you have any questions?"

"Not really. The fake conversations are very annoying. Do people really talk like that?"

"I don't know. Katie said the same thing."

"Well, some of it is really stupid."

"It's not a bad book, though; it's got some good information in between those conversations."

"I guess."

"Do you understand all the changes that are going to happen—like starting your period?" I took another bite of my crispy bacon.

"Mom, I already know all about that from Karen and Katie. And I don't really want to talk about it. That stuff is private." She poured a few more drops of hot sauce onto her potatoes.

"Yes, it's private, but it's also normal and something we shouldn't be afraid to discuss. You can talk about these changes with me or with your sisters or with your youth leader. The changes that occur as you become a woman are nothing to be ashamed of."

"I know."

We ate silently for a few minutes. Then my heart began to pound as fear and shame threatened to overcome my courage to talk about my past actions toward Kelly. After a few moments, my courage returned like the sun after a passing thunderstorm.

"Well, I have something important and private that we need to talk about back in the room after we finish breakfast."

"Okay."

When we got back into the room, she grabbed the book and flopped on her stomach on the bed, feet in the air.

"What is it, Mom?"

I got down on my knees next to the bed, took the book out of her hands and set it on the bed. I clasped her hands in mine as I began my confession.

"Kelly, I need to ask you to forgive me."

"Forgive you for what?"

"Do you remember when you were almost three and I threw you across the room into a pile of blankets?"

"Not really."

"Well, I remember it. I was very angry with your dad and I took it out on you. I was wrong to do it and I am asking you to forgive me."

"Mom, don't cry."

She took one of her hands out of my grasp and smoothed over the top of my head as if she were petting a much-loved dog.

I sobbed into the bedspread for what seemed like an eternity.

Pull yourself together! Your sobbing is just going to make things worse. You need to be the strong one. Remember, you are *the mom.*

"I'm really sorry, Kelly; I never meant to hurt you."

"I know, Mom. I forgive you."

"Kelly, you know I love you very much and you are very special. You are such a gift to me—the best birthday present a mom could ask for! I hate it that I hurt you. Even though you don't remember it right now, it means so much to me that you forgive me."

Reflection. It was hard to ask Kelly to forgive me, but it felt really important. I was afraid that my episode of abuse had somehow made her feel rejected or insecure. And I was afraid that sense of rejection would cause her to seek acceptance and security through sexual promiscuity, as I believed I had done. The first testimony I wrote in college about my conversion experience told this narrative—that my parents' divorce and my father's absence led me to look for love in all the wrong places, and that I finally found it in Christ. While there is much truth in that story, I've since come to realize that my story of faith is far more complicated and the reasons I chose to have sex before marriage were also more complicated. Unfortunately, that redemption narrative inspired fear in me—what if I did something wrong as a parent that caused my children to go looking for love in all the wrong places?

#facingthetalk: Examine your own story and identify areas where you experience the most shame. Be honest about your failings and consider how to seek forgiveness.

Pay attention to things that are difficult to talk about. Look at your relationship with your spouse as well as your child. Take responsibility for things you have done wrong in your relationship with your daughter.

Shame says, "I am a terrible person." Guilt says, "I did something wrong." Don't give in to the feeling that admission of guilt is a sign of weakness. We all do wrong things. Trying to hide the things we've done wrong perpetuates systems of shame. And when you're hiding behind a barrier of shame, it's difficult to bond. It's difficult to talk about important things like sex, love and relationships. These getaways are prime times to repair significant rifts in your relationship with your daughter.

Kelly didn't consciously remember my abusive behavior, so she may not have fully understood what she was forgiving me for. But I choose to trust her forgiveness. I also understand that forgiveness is a process. I hope that if memories surface, Kelly won't be afraid to talk to someone about them. I hope she will learn to understand the complexities of love and grace. I hope she will know that she is loved and accepted fully.

How-To Sex Talk No. 4

We almost didn't make it. The flyer came home announcing sex ed classes at school for Kimberly and I still hadn't taken her on her special weekend getaway! We got the flyer in January. Fortunately, Kimberly's midwinter break overlapped with my February trip to Portland, so I was able to make it work. I booked our train tickets, and the planning of the last How-To getaway began.

"All aboard!" Kimberly, age ten, held my hand as we wheeled our suitcases toward the train headed for Portland.

I was never one of those moms who cried when she sent her kids off to their first day of kindergarten, but I was feeling a bit sentimental about this getaway with my youngest daughter. She was so innocent, so young. Especially when compared with her older sisters. As our train departed for Portland, it felt like the last vestiges of childhood innocence would soon be slipping away.

We arrived in Centralia, Washington, the halfway point between Seattle and Portland, and walked across the street to the Olympic Club Hotel and Theater. The Olympic Club was formerly a "gentleman's" establishment dating back to the early nineteen hundreds.

"Mom, can we go to the movie here in the hotel tonight?" Kimberly sat on the edge of the bed brushing her long hair.

"Mmm, dinner and a movie. That sounds like fun. Let's see what's playing."

She found the schedule on the nightstand and announced excitedly, "*Twilight*! *Twilight* is playing! Mom, can we go?"

I had already seen *Twilight* with Katie on opening night. The older girls were hooked on the young adult vampire series, and while I didn't always have time to keep up with the books they were reading, I tried to at least go see the movies. Movies like *Twilight* opened many doors for stimulating conversations about faith and culture.

"Sure, that sounds like a great idea. What time is it playing?"

"The next show starts at six o'clock."

"Great, that gives us a couple of hours to start our sex talk and then we can eat dinner at the movie."

I had left the *How You Are Changing* book at home this time, deciding to use some online resources and try to be a little more conversational with Kimberly. I knew she'd probably heard a lot of the details from her sisters.

We chatted about God's good plan for sex between a man and woman and how babies are good gifts from God. I pulled up a website with some specifics on how reproduction works and set the laptop on her lap.

I used a resource from the Washington State Department of Education Family Life and Sexual Health (FLASH) curriculum for consistency since that was the curriculum her school would be using. I hoped it would help her connect the ideas she would hear at school with what we discussed on our getaway.

I got a book out of my suitcase and sat next to her on the bed.

After reading for a bit, Kimberly brushed her overgrown bangs out of her blue eyes and looked up at me from the computer screen.

"So you and Dad had sex four times?"

I peeked at the computer screen to see that she had just finished reading the section on how the sperm meets the egg.

While Kimberly sometimes struggled with math, she had this equation all figured out: having sex equals making a baby. Four babies equals four times having sex.

I was tempted to allow her concrete thinking to remain unchallenged. Perhaps if she believed that every instance of sex resulted in a baby, she would be more likely to wait until she wanted a baby to have sex. But I knew others would tell her the truth. And I wanted to be the first one to tell her this truth.

I put my arm around her shoulders and looked more closely at the pictures of the sperm and the egg.

"Well, the sperm and the egg don't meet each other every time people have sex." I stroked her long hair because she still let me; it was soft and comforting and reminded me of when my mom used to play with my hair.

While I wanted Kimberly to believe she could get pregnant every time she had sex, she needed to know that conception is far more complicated. People who want to conceive can't and others who shouldn't conceive do. A part of me was tempted to go into my spiel about how sex is for bonding and expressing love, not just for procreation, but it didn't feel like the right time.

"Go on and read the next section; it might explain things a little more." We snuggled a little closer on the bed as we returned to our reading.

While I was still sometimes nervous and fearful when talking with my girls about sex, by my fourth round I had become convinced that these weekend getaways were more about bonding than information sharing. The greatest truth I could convey was that she was loved. The second greatest truth? There was no shame in talking about sex and she didn't have to fear the changes her body was about to experience in full force.

"What's next?" She closed the laptop and set it at the bottom of the bed.

"Well, do you have any more questions?"

"Not really. It all sounds kind of gross with the swapping of fluids and stuff. And penises are just weird-looking!"

"I know! They're all wrinkly and change shape and size. It's quite strange. But it's not gross. It's just a normal body part for boys. Most boys probably think vaginas are weird too. Someday you might learn to appreciate such things."

"Eeew. I don't want to think about that. Let's talk about something else." She rested her head on my chest as if settling in for a good, long snuggle.

"Why do boys like boobs so much?"

"Great question. Maybe that's something you can ask your dad about. I'm not sure all boys think boobs are attractive. Some boys find a girl's bottom attractive, others like long legs, and some prefer smart girls while others prefer sporty girls. Everyone is attracted to different features."

We snuggled and chatted for a while longer before she asked, "Is it time to go to the movie yet?"

"Yes, it's almost time. Let's head downstairs in five minutes."

We arrived early and picked the comfiest couch near the front of the theater. She saved my spot while I went to the counter and ordered our dinner. The theater was a cozy and casual place where it felt like we were sitting in our own living room watching a movie with friends. Our dinner was served a few minutes before the movie started.

"Mom, are you on Team Jacob or Team Edward?" she asked after licking the ketchup off her pinky finger.

"I'm on Team Bella. I support her right to choose."

The *Twilight* series revolves around the classic love triangle theme. And Bella is the beauty caught in the middle of an epic struggle between two dangerously alluring men, one a vampire, the other a werewolf.

One of my favorite scenes is when Edward, the vampire, attempts to kiss Bella for the first time. He has already explained

how irresistible her scent is to him and how he has chosen a
lifestyle of refusing to drink human blood.

He magically arrives in her bedroom and sits on the end of
Bella's bed facing her. After a few seconds of dialogue Edward
leans in.

"I just wanna try one thing. Stay very still," he says, then very
slowly moves in for the kiss.

Bella's breath quickens and she begins to shift slightly in his
direction.

"No, don't move."

After what seems like endless moments, their lips finally meet.

He kisses her, and she kisses him back.

She climbs on his lap, moving as the aggressor, as she forcefully kisses his too-red lips.

Quickly he turns on her and nearly pins her to the bed, then
flies off with his vampire superspeed ability, slamming himself
backward into the wall.

"Stop!" His command seems more directed at himself than
at Bella.

"I'm sorry," Bella timidly replies.

He drops his shoulders as if relaxing from a fight-or-flight
situation.

"I'm stronger than I thought," Edward says.

"Yeah, I wish I could say the same."

"I can't ever lose control with you." Edward turns to leave.

"Hey, don't go."

The scene ends with haunting music while Edward watches
Bella sleep.

I had already discussed this scene with my older girls. While
I may not like all the ideas such a scene represents, I knew I
could use it to present an idea that was important for them to

consider. As we left the theater, I prepared to give my "Bella and Edward's First Kiss" speech later that night.

"So what did you think of the movie? Was it as good as you hoped?" We were back in our room but not quite ready for bed.

"Yep. It was good. But that scene near the end when Bella freaked out and said she couldn't live without Edward was really bad. And Edward always looked like he was in pain when he was kissing her—that seemed weird."

"I agree. The kissing scenes are kind of awkward. But their first kiss? That's something worth thinking about."

"Which one was that?"

"The one in her bedroom when he flies off of her."

"Oh, that one."

"Well, if there's ever a boy who tries to kiss you and tells you he just can't stop himself, you remember Edward. He stopped himself and he's not even human. He's a vampire! Any boy who says he can't stop is just lying."

"Mom! It's just a movie. And I don't plan on kissing any boys anytime soon."

"I know, I know. I'm just sayin'. We all have a choice about who we kiss and how we kiss. If you tell someone to stop, they should always stop. And if they don't, you should talk to someone about it. You can always talk to me, your dad, your sisters or your youth leader."

"Okay, Mom. I get it. Can we go to bed now?"

We put on our PJs, slid under the covers and snuggled one last time before we drifted off to peaceful sleep.

Reflection. I knew Kimberly would probably never ask her dad why boys liked boobs. And the introvert in him would never volunteer such information. Sometimes physical attraction is beyond understanding. And that's a good thing since most of us

don't look like the magazine cover girls men are supposed to be
attracted to. The reality is, most of us are attracted to more than
one person in our lifetime, and we're attracted to them for different reasons. While physical attraction is a part of most relationships, it is not the most important part. I don't believe in the
idea of a singular, fated attraction often called a "soulmate," nor
do I think it's healthy to imagine a kind of strong attraction that
leads someone to say "I can't live without you" as Bella declared
in *Twilight*. But I decided not to go into the details of all my
theories of attraction on this getaway. I knew there would be
plenty of other opportunities.

Some of my friends avoided the *Twilight* series because it
featured vampires; others argued that it sexualized violence. But
most of my friends jumped on the *Twilight* train and rode it all
the way to the end. I went along for the ride, but I refused to
pick sides. Instead, I used it as an opportunity to talk with my
girls about faith and culture in a way that was relevant to them.

#facingthetalk: Learn to ask good questions but don't be afraid to
have a few prepared speeches as well. You might be surprised to find
that a question your girl asks opens the door for you to say something
you've thought through carefully ahead of time.

As I think back over these four getaways, I notice that I had
more anxiety with my first and third daughters than with my
second and fourth. I am in the process of development as much
as they are. It's important to recognize that there is no blueprint
for these talks. We are each unique and have our own fears to face
and relationship struggles to work through. Sometimes it's harder
than others. But even amidst the struggle, it's always worth it. I
enjoyed each getaway and cherish the memories shared.

Talking Topics

Ages Nine to Twelve

W hen my husband picked Katie up from Sunday school, Teacher Lanny pulled him aside. Lanny was concerned about Katie's attire. That warm summer Sunday she was wearing an ankle-length, light-blue spaghetti-strap dress that came with a cap-sleeved lace jacket. But that Sunday, like many other days, she had decided not to wear the jacket. The light-blue dress brought out the blue in her eyes. She looked like a china doll. But Teacher Lanny saw something different. He told Ken that Katie's bare shoulders were a problem and that she should cover up in the future. She was five years old.

Modesty

At this stage of our parenting, Ken and I had to divide and conquer to manage our kids in our large megachurch. My husband picked up the two older girls from Sunday school, while I headed to the nursery to gather our baby and toddler. After we found each other in what's called the "mallway" of our church, Katie seemed a little less excited than usual to tell me about her Sunday school craft. She clung to my side as Kelly ran to greet her daddy.

Katie was not usually the clingy type, so I knew something was up. She hung her head as I stroked her curls and shot my husband an inquisitive look. With a slightly exasperated tone, my husband explained her downcast demeanor by telling me what the Sunday school teacher had said. I tried to hide my annoyance, not really knowing what to think and wondering when bare little-girl shoulders had become a problem. I put my hand on Katie's shoulder and it seemed as if the shame spread from her to me in one great surge, submerging me in my own pool.

Unfortunately, my annoyance and shame got misdirected. I curtly asked my little girl, "What happened to your jacket? Why didn't you wear it to church today?"

Later that evening, I watched my three oldest girls laugh and splash in the tub. As I helped them get clean, I tickled their tummies, wrapped them in their Lion King hoodie towels and began the bedtime routine. Their favorite lullaby, by consensus, was "the 'pecial song." I had a diverse repertoire of lullabies, including multiple verses of "Twinkle, Twinkle," but this was the most frequently requested. I've even had occasion to sing it to them in their teen years!

My husband and I were snuggling in bed after I nursed Kimberly, and I asked, "I wonder what Teacher Lanny's problem was? That must have been kind of creepy to have him talk to you about our daughter's bare shoulders."

I crawled into my favorite place, resting my head on his broad shoulder. He wrapped his arm around me and caressed my shoulder, answering, "Yeah, it was weird. I don't think we need to worry about it, though. It's not like Katie did anything wrong."

"But it's frustrating. Our girls are so young and so cute—are bare shoulders really a problem?" I felt a sense of peace and oneness as Ken's fingers gently moved up and down my arm.

"Well, apparently in church they are. Let's not make a big deal out of it." I kissed him on the cheek and closed my eyes, drifting off to sleep in the comfort of his embrace.

My husband, the peacemaker, often helps diffuse my annoyance. But I wonder if perhaps we should have been more annoyed at Teacher Lanny. I'm sad that my annoyance got misplaced onto my daughter. It wasn't her fault that Teacher Lanny sexualized her appearance. Bare shoulders don't always lead to sexual intercourse, even between married couples.

Reflection. "The 'pecial song" was one of my favorites too. It communicated what I believed to be true—we are very special, each one of us handmade by God to praise him all our days. It's not just our hearts, our spirits or our voices that praise God, but our very presence in bodies with skin on. I wanted my girls to know that their bodies were nothing to be ashamed of. All of God's creation is good, including five-year-old-girl shoulders.

You may be wondering why I've included this story in a chapter about nine- to twelve-year-olds. It's because I didn't develop my ideas of modesty in isolation or all of the sudden when my daughters reached a certain age. My ideas about modesty were shaped and formed by my experiences growing up, by my church community and by the popular media culture.

As you think about how you might have responded to this situation, reflect on your own story. What's had the most influence on your ideas about modesty? Is it your family culture and upbringing? Are you reacting against popular media culture? What messages about modesty do you experience in your church community? How would you respond if this happened when your daughter was seven or ten? What about age thirteen or after your daughter began developing breasts and hips? Who decides when and whether showing a little skin is a problem? Who told this forty-something male Sunday school teacher that bare five-year-old-girl shoulders were a problem? Who was it a problem for? The five-year-old boys in the class or the teacher?

When I was five, I was still taking baths with my four-year-old boy cousin and nobody thought twice about us being naked together in the tub at grandma's house. There was an innocence and asexuality about our preschool bodies. Even after entering elementary school, most boys and girls don't think of each other in sexually objectifying ways. Sure, I had a crush on a boy in second grade and thought he was cute, but our language for those experiences was much different than the language children use today. Our interest was marked more by the normal curiosity of developing children who are trying to navigate what it means to be a boy or a girl in society.

Today, by the time our girls reach the age of nine or ten, they are likely to have been exposed to many images of sexualized girl bodies. From the ten-inch Bratz fashion dolls wearing fishnet tights, which outsold Barbie dolls in 2006, to the 2010 viral video of seven-year-old girls dressed in sexy lingerie and gyrating to Beyonce's "All the Single Ladies," the sexualization of girlhood has become pervasive. The messages our girls receive about their role in the world, even at this young age, is that their value and power are in their sexuality. Our initial reaction may be a desire to shelter them from these influences, but the ubiquity of sexual messages would require us to move into a convent or onto a deserted island in order to avoid them.

"Increasingly over the past 10 years, we've seen an escalation in the sexualization of young girls," says developmental psychologist Deborah Tolman. "There's an inappropriate imposition of sexuality on young girls, and, as girls enter adolescence, they're learning to sexualize themselves."[1] Diane Levin and Jean Kilbourne, authors of So Sexy So Soon, are deeply worried about the price children pay for the sexualization of their childhood. "Girls and boys constantly encounter sexual messages and images that they cannot understand and that can confuse and frighten them. A narrow definition of femininity and sexuality encourages girls to focus heavily on appearance and sex appeal. They learn at a very young age that their value is determined by how beautiful, thin, 'hot,' and sexy they are."[2]

The primary message communicated through the media is that women exist for the pleasure and consumption of men—they are objects to be possessed, owned and used to fulfill male needs, desires and dreams. Adolescent and pre-adolescent boys are one of the largest markets for some of the more extreme versions of this message, as illustrated in the Media Education Foundation documentary film *Dreamworlds 3*, which helps viewers understand the influence of music videos and pop culture and the dangerously narrow set of myths about sex and gender that those videos portray. The documentary inspires viewers to reflect critically on images and ideas that they might otherwise ignore as unimportant or just entertainment.[3] Unfortunately, boys and young men who attend church and go to youth groups are not immune from the influence of these dreamworlds.

Faith communities have responded to the oversexualization and objectification of women in many different ways. For some this response has been an intensification of modesty rules, which teach girls to cover up their sexy bodies because the media is right; their bodies are sexual and therefore dangerous for boys' visual consumption. The subtle message is that girls should be ashamed of their bodies and that they are responsible for boys' and men's lustful looks. But as Emily Maynard, a Portland blogger writing for ChurchLeaders, says, "I don't think dressing according to a set of modesty rules will ever stop another person from lusting."[4]

While teaching our girls to dress appropriately in unassuming ways is important, strict modesty rules and the "modest is hottest" messages are doing more harm than good by setting up equally unrealistic and unattainable ideals. These modesty ideals are merely the flip side of the media objectification of women. Sharon Hodde Miller notes in a *Christianity Today* article, "The Christian rhetoric of modesty, rather than offering believers an alternative to the sexual objectification of women, often continues the objectification, just in a different form."[5]

A weekend getaway introducing our girls to normal sexual development and helping them understand what sexual intercourse is all about is necessary and can facilitate healthy bonding, but they need much more than this. Our girls need us to be a faithful presence in their lives. I've heard it said that as the body of Christ, we are like Jesus with skin on. We need to be available to help our girls process these often confusing and frightening messages, and we need to offer alternative messages about their bodies and their developing selves.

> **#facingthetalk:** Don't shame girls for being exposed to sexual messages. It happens every day. Ask what they think. Empower them to think well.
>
> Continue the conversations started on the weekend getaway. Intentionally listen to pop music, watch the movies and TV shows they are watching with them on occasion, and pay attention to the conversations they have with their friends from school. Be careful about shaming them for hearing about, talking about or being exposed to sexual messages and images. It's unavoidable. Shaming them for being exposed to things they are not in control of only gives more power to those messages.

Our girls are exposed to sexual messages from a very early age, and these messages seem to intensify around ages nine to twelve. From ages five to twelve, one of a child's primary developmental tasks, according to Erikson's stages of psychosocial development, is asking, "Can I make it in the world of people and things?" Competence is a big issue at this stage. Our girls are asking themselves in subconscious ways, "Am I smart enough? Am I strong enough? Am I friendly enough?" With the sexualization of childhood, our girls are asking a new question: "Am I sexy enough?" In the next psychosocial stage, their primary task is identity development. They ask, "Who am I, and what can I be?" As our girls make this transition, I wonder how this focus on sexualization impacts their identity development. What can we do to mitigate the harmful effects of the sexualization of girlhood?

As children develop, they wrestle with questions of power. Between three and six years old, they learn to exert power to affect relationships, and they learn the effects of power by observing and setting up power struggles. These questions of power continue in the six- to twelve-year stage, when girls focus on the structures of family and the world around them. The sexual messages they are exposed to give them a sense that their power is found in their appearance, their attractiveness, their degree of "hotness."

As our girls take in these messages, some subtly desire this power while others fear it. Each of my girls responded differently to these messages. There were often intrafamilial power struggles over what kind of clothes they chose to wear as they experimented with power in their extrafamilial relationships. And these dynamics were not always about attracting boys. Sometimes they were more about rivalry with other girls and seeking acceptance among peers. When we focus on worrying about modesty in relation to sex appeal, we often miss other important aspects of girl culture that shape and form our daughters.

Modesty Rules

My first time in the juniors department at the local department store was an adventure. At age twelve Karen had outgrown girls' clothes and was blossoming into a beautiful young lady. As she tried on a few outfits, I noticed a shift in how she evaluated her clothes. When she was younger it was all about function—she was active and picked clothes that fit her activities. Even when she was choosing a dress, it had to be one that twirled. Not so much because it was pretty, but because it moved with her as she spun. Now I saw her look in the mirror with a much more critical eye and greater level of self-awareness.

I wanted desperately for her to not worry about her looks. I wanted to help her develop a healthy body image. I wanted her to know that she was lovely and lovable no matter how her body shape changed over time. But I had no idea where to begin. Each time she tried on a top that showed a little skin, this tape kept running in my head—*will she get in trouble if she wears that to church?* After her younger sister was told to cover up, those thoughts kept popping up in my mind.

Both the media culture and the church culture are telling girls that their bodies have magical power over boys. The images in magazines and movies tell them they can get whatever boy they want if they're hot enough. The modesty rules in church tell them they can make boys lust after them and cause them to sin if they're too hot. Both tell the same story as flip sides of the same coin—girl bodies are powerful, but only in a sexual way.

Unfortunately, I swallowed the modesty rules hook, line and sinker.

• • •

"Are you going to the neighborhood barbecue?" I asked as Karen entered the kitchen where I was mashing the avocados for guacamole.

"Yes, I'm going to head down now with Katie," she replied.

"Not like that you aren't!"

"Why? What's wrong?" She looked down at the V-neck on her T-shirt that plunged practically to her belly button. Okay, that's an exaggeration. But that's what it seemed like in the moment.

"That shirt is way too low-cut. You don't want the neighbor boys staring at your boobs, do you?" I mashed the avocados a little more forcefully as I imagined not only the neighbor boys but the neighbor men ogling my daughter's breasts.

"No, of course not! But Mom, this is what all the girls are wearing. It's really not that bad." She pulled up the neckline just a little.

I was not so easily appeased.

"You go put on a tank top under that shirt before you go to the barbecue or you can stay home." My Love and Logic parenting ideals were being squelched by my anxiety over modesty rules.

"I don't have a tank top that matches. And seriously, Mom, it's not like there are going to be many people there. It's all people we know."

"I told you what you need to do. Please stop arguing." The avocados were completely mashed and it was time to add the rest of the ingredients.

"Whatever." She whirled out of the room and stomped down the stairs to her bedroom to change.

I got out the lemon juice, hoping to give the guacamole just the right bite of tartness. But the sour taste in my mouth made it hard for me to judge.

Reflection. I came up with some pretty strict modesty rules in our home for a while. I hoped these rules would protect my girls from male ogling. But low necklines don't make men lecherous. It's not my daughters' fault that some men have excessive, offensive or inappropriate sexual desires. Some women find men gawking at them no matter what they're wearing. Should we tell attractive women to change their body shape or the size of their lips just because some men might be tempted to stare?

We live in a highly anxious society where 20 percent of women have experienced sexual abuse as a child.[6] Is it any wonder we're anxious for our girls? If it didn't happen to you, I suspect you know someone who experienced unwanted touch, indecent exposure, even rape. But that doesn't mean all men and adolescent boys are potential perpetrators and all women and girls are potential victims. Helping our girls understand that some men are dangerous, but not all, may reduce our anxiety. We can teach them how to defend themselves if attacked without blaming them for asking for it by the way they dress.

Nobody asks to be raped. Even women who are dressed modestly are raped. Sometimes men are raped. Sexual violence is a real concern for parents, but it can happen no matter how we try to prevent it. Let's empower our girls to get help from safe people when they feel threatened. Shaming them for the clothes they wear disempowers them and sets them up as both victim and perpetrator in the sexual crime drama, letting men off the hook for their lustful and abusive behavior.

It may feel uncomfortable to imagine having these conversations with your daughter at such a young age, but these conversations are important even if you don't think your daughter is influenced by the oversexualization of girls. I didn't have these kinds of conversations with my first daughter right away; it wasn't until she was older that I recognized how much fear I had surrounding this topic and how much shame I was communicating to her.

#facingthetalk: Don't tell girls it's their fault when boys fantasize or men lust. Encourage them to talk to a trusted adult when they feel uncomfortable.

Confront your own anxiety about sexual violence before talking to your girls about it. Help them to be aware of how others view their bodies and give them the tools to make wise choices about what to wear and what not to wear. Trust them to make wise choices. Teach them to speak up when they feel others are looking at them inappropriately. Pay attention to the ways they feel shame or blame for boys' fantasies and men's lust. Teach them how to find safe ways of escape when they feel threatened.

Once she became an adult I shared with her some of my experiences with sexual abuse and how that shaped my early parenting.

See appendix B on sexual abuse and violence against women for more resources in this area.

What the Bible Says About Lust and Causing Others to Stumble

When Jesus talked about lust, he didn't shame or blame anyone for being a stumbling block by virtue of their physical appearance, like the woman caught in adultery in John 8. I've often wondered about this woman. Why was she the only one brought before Jesus? Where was the man she was committing adultery with? Were the religious leaders blaming the woman for the man's lust?

Jesus foiled their attempts at shaming and blaming by sticking to his corrective to the law offered in the Sermon on the Mount:

> "You have heard that it was said, 'You shall not commit adultery.' But I tell you that anyone who looks at a woman lustfully has already committed adultery with her in his heart. If your right eye causes you to stumble, gouge it out

and throw it away. It is better for you to lose one part of your body than for your whole body to be thrown into hell. And if your right hand causes you to stumble, cut it off and throw it away. It is better for you to lose one part of your body than for your whole body to go into hell." (Matthew 5:27-30)

Jesus doesn't say, "If you look lustfully at a woman, tell her to cover up better so she won't cause you to stumble." He squarely puts the responsibility for lust on the person doing the lusting, not the person being lusted after. Shouldn't we do the same?

Jesus' injunction about not causing others to stumble, found in Matthew 18 and Mark 9, follows on the heels of conversations with people who desire positions of power. His caution about stumbling blocks is directed toward those who would prevent young believers from coming directly to Jesus, who would hinder their childlike faith with roadblocks of religious rules and regulations, like the ones the Pharisees had set up. Elaborate purity codes and ideals of perfection communicate that only certain people have access to God. Jesus shows us that we all have access to God's love and forgiveness through him. Showing too much cleavage or a belly button does not result in the proverbial millstone being hung around a neck.

But that's not what our modesty rules tell our girls.

When we talk to our girls about modesty, we need to be careful to help them to understand that men are responsible for their own lust. They are responsible for how they use their power—including the power of sexual attraction. Ask your girl to think about why she chooses certain clothes. Is it to be attractive? Is it to be comfortable? Remember that at this stage of development our girls are asking, "Can I make it in the world of people and things?" And in many ways they're hearing that the only way to "make it" is to be attractive. So it's important to talk about attraction; it plays a significant part in girls' clothing choices. If we bring attraction to a place of awareness and discussion, we empower our girls to make wise choices. Are they trying to exert power through the way they dress—to make others love and accept them more? Who are they trying to please with their clothing choices?

Having honest conversations with our girls about clothes that expose part of their bodies—their breasts, for example—is a good place to start empowering them to make wise choices. Ask them why they want to wear clothes that show cleavage. Invite them to honestly examine whether they're looking for attention or hoping to impress their female friends with their fashionableness or their male friends with their sexiness. Ask them how it makes them feel when others look at their breasts. Teach them to think about unconscious motivations that may be influenced by their desire for friends' approval or other emotional needs. Guide them to set their own boundaries as they get older; this teaches them that they are responsible for their own bodies. Some women choose to cover up not because modest is hottest, or to prevent men from raping them, but because it demonstrates a healthy respect for personal privacy and a resistance to the objectifying forces of an oversexualized culture.

It would be nice if we could tell our girls that the only person they need to worry about pleasing with their choice of clothing is Jesus, but it's just not that simple. We should help them know how Jesus loves and accepts them no matter what they wear, no matter what shape or size their body is, and no matter what others think about them. But the truth is, what others think about them matters. And often it's what other girls think about them that matters most. When we talk about modesty in sexual terms, we overlook a powerful dynamic—the dynamic of imitation and rivalry.

René Girard, a sociologist and theologian, says that all desire is borrowed desire.[7] We tend to desire things because others desire them. We look to others as our models and then imitate them. This imitation leads to rivalry and eventually violence. He suggests that the way out of this system of rivalry and violence is to look to Jesus as our ultimate model.

As parents and as the body of Christ we can inspire our girls to choose Jesus as their model as we imitate Christ. One of the ways we imitate Christ is by showing unconditional love and acceptance of our daughters.

> **#facingthetalk:** Are our girls trying to make others love them more by the way they dress? Love them unconditionally, no matter what they wear. Teach them to be responsible for examining whether they're trying to make others love them more by the way they dress. Ask them who their role models are. Help them choose godly role models who imitate Christ. It's tempting to teach them that they are responsible if a man lusts after them because of the way they dress, but resist this temptation. We are all responsible for our own choices. Help them to choose Christ.

Teaching our girls healthy boundaries in this area is important. And healthy boundaries involve a balance between freedom and responsibility. Freedom is the ability to make choices out of a sense of what is valuable and important, not out of fear or shame or rivalry. When our girls choose their clothes out of freedom, they're more likely to choose clothes that reflect who they are, clothes that are right for them, clothes they wholeheartedly enjoy wearing. Responsibility is the ability to exert power and make choices in ways that are healthy and loving, ways that consider others as important. But responsibility also means being able to discern what they are not responsible for, like men's lust. We need to teach them how to say no to harmful or inappropriate behavior. Teaching our daughters healthy boundaries involves helping them know where their responsibility ends and others' begins.

Preparing for Periods

"Mom, will you talk to Dad for me?" Karen, age twelve, had already finished packing for her YMCA father-daughter trip to Camp Orkila and her duffle bag was at the bottom of the pile in the back of the Volvo station wagon.

"Why? What's up?"

"Well, last year Bridget started her period on one of these camping trips and it kinda freaked her out. Her dad was not prepared."

"Oh my, that must have been awkward. Of course I'll talk with your dad and make sure he's prepared. Do you have those pads they gave you in sex ed class at school?"

"I don't know where I put them. They might be in my closet or under my bed. I don't remember."

I wasn't interested in beginning a treasure hunt in her jungle of a bedroom, so I headed to my bathroom to look for supplies. I found an old makeup bag that was the perfect size and offered complete concealment. I zipped up a few pads and tampons in the bag and headed for the garage.

"Dear, we need to talk before you leave for Camp Orkila." Ken was putting the sleeping bags into the car.

"What's up?" He squished down the last sleeping bag so he'd be able to see out of the rearview mirror.

"Nothing. It's just a girl thing we need to talk about. I heard that Bridget started her period on one of these campouts and I don't want you to be unprepared. Karen could start her period any day now."

"Great. Can't she just pack some girlie stuff?" He gently closed the hatch on the Volvo.

"Sure, but her bag is on the bottom of the pile and you know how easily she loses things. I think it would be better to keep some supplies in the glove box. It's helpful for you to know about these things anyway. It'll make it easier if any of our girls start their period while they're with you."

Ken is the second of two sons with no sisters. I doubt his mother talked about her menstrual cycle in front of her boys. In many ways this was all new territory for him.

"Okay, fine. What do I need to do?"

Ken was never one to give in to stereotypes or treat our girls as if they were incapable of doing most things boys could do, but he drew the line at talking about periods. There were some things that would always remain in the girl domain no matter how committed he was to growing strong daughters.

"Here's a bag with supplies that should fit in the glove box. Young girls can get really self-conscious about their period, so if Karen asks you to go get it for her, please don't ask questions or make any public announcements. Just get the bag and do whatever she asks without making a big deal of it."

"All right." He took the bag between forefinger and thumb, holding it like it had cooties, and carefully put it in the glove box.

I went back inside to find Karen and let her know the deal was done. Her dad was prepared. She didn't need to be afraid.

Reflection. It was important for me to facilitate bonding between my girls and Ken. After all, I'd been told as a young Christian that my sexual promiscuity was the result of a "father wound." A father wound is harm caused by a father through his active negative influence (abuse), passive negative influence (emotional absence) or actual physical absence (fatherlessness). I was still resolving issues that had emerged as a result of my father's abusive behavior and subsequent absence from my life after my parents divorced. Unfortunately my fear often provoked me to take a controlling and manipulative stance toward my husband rather than seeking a cooperative relationship.

I was thankful when Ken took the girls on camping trips. The YMCA father-daughter program offered structured experiences that encouraged bonding. But as the girls began to transition into puberty, it became more awkward for him to stay connected with them. And I became a bit more anxious and controlling. I've since learned to recognize my fear and let his relationship with the girls develop naturally according to his parenting style, not mine.

Sometimes a disconnect between fathers and daughters occurs because fathers feel unprepared, uncomfortable, uninformed and unable to identify with the changes their girls are experiencing. The reality is, most mothers are charged with the task of informing both their girls and the men in their lives about the changes that are happening at this stage of development. And it's not an easy task.

Some dads are better at bonding during the pre-adolescent years and some are better at bonding with teens. I struggled the most with bonding during the pre-adolescent years and bonded more during the teen years. For Ken it was the reverse. Strong parental bonds with both parents have been identified as positive influences in the lives of girls who choose to wait until later to have sex. It's never too early or too late to bond with your girls. Early bonds last a long time. Even if it seems there is a

#facingthetalk: Even though it's awkward, fathers who acknowledge and are not afraid to talk to their girls about periods help remove shame from the subject. Fathers, pay attention to your comfort level and your girls' comfort level when talking about periods and other normal developmental processes that are unique to girls. Mothers, talk with your girls about including their dad in conversations about the changes they're experiencing. Talk with your husband about the awkward feelings he might be experiencing—this helps minimize shame and fear. Invite participation at a level he feels comfortable with. Be careful not to oversexualize the changes in your girls. And don't be afraid to have a few conversations in the presence of brothers. Talking about changes only in gender-separated spaces may reinforce shame over sexual differences.

My counselor offered me an important distinction between secrecy and privacy that has helped me talk with my girls and their father about sensitive topics. Secrecy and hiding often lead to feelings of shame and disconnection. Privacy and discretion encourage healthy boundaries that lead to feelings of self-confidence and safety. Refusing to talk about normal things like periods and puberty often shrouds the topic in secrecy and shame. Acknowledging that it's a very personal and private topic helps remove the shame and sets the stage for negotiating appropriate family boundaries for when and how these topics are discussed.

disconnect during the transition to puberty or during the teen years, rest assured, your love will not be forgotten.

Adolescence is a time of intense transition. There is nothing stable, predictable or reasonable about it. We try to understand it and seek to know what's normal, what's typical, what's right. We measure it in stages and put boundaries around it with time. We look for signs and try to prepare ourselves for what's next. I thought I was ready for this transition, but the process of maturation and differentiation into adult human beings was far more complex than I'd ever imagined. At times it felt very chaotic—especially the first time.

I remember the chaos of my own transition from childhood

to adulthood all too well. When we think of chaos, we often associate it with complete disorder and utter confusion. We fear it and even sing in our worship songs about how thankful we are that God brings order out of chaos. And while it's true that God does bring order out of chaos, that doesn't mean life is predictable or orderly in the ways we desire. God's order is higher than ours.

Chaos theory helps me understand God's order in new ways. Chaos theory tells us that at the heart of what appears to be unpredictable and random lies a hidden and beautiful order. Margaret Wheatley writes in *Leadership and the New Science: Discovering Order in a Chaotic World*, "Chaos has always partnered with order—a concept that contradicts our common definition of chaos—but until we could see it with computers, we saw only turbulence, energy without predictable form."[8] Adolescence may be turbulent at times, and the unpredictability of it may feel overwhelming, but I am learning to think of the chaos of adolescence in more positive terms. I think of chaos as unpredictability governed by grace.

A chaotic system is a complex, dynamic system that is extremely sensitive to initial input. Genetic factors, early childhood experiences and social setting are all significant initial inputs into the development of identity. But like many complex dynamic systems, identity formation often goes through a turbulent and seemingly chaotic phase before the beautiful patterns of a person's unique existence emerge. For some, the chaos is mostly experienced on the inside—they continue along in the family system with what seems like only minor turbulence affecting those around them. For others the transition is experienced as a series of storms sending the family system into a state of emergency.

The process of forming an identity involves creating a coherent sense of self as a person in relation to others and the world. And this process ramps up to a whole new level at adolescence. It's a challenging task for a girl to make sense of the multitude of physical, emotional and social changes in the context of her ever-expanding worldview. And it doesn't stop at the end of adolescence—there's not one moment in any woman's life when she fully knows herself. Rather, her identity evolves throughout adulthood, building on the competencies of childhood and adolescence. But once a person's identity goes through the chaos of adolescence, patterns do tend to appear. The adult that emerges from adolescence looks quite different from the little girl who once twirled around the living room in a dress floating on air. But some pieces of that little girl will always remain.

Where Did My Little Girl Go?

*T*hirteen-year-old Karen was spending more and more time alone in her room, so when I found her reading on her bed, I took the opportunity to spill my guts to her privately. I plopped down next to her with a heavy sigh.

"Karen, I need to explain something to you." I propped myself up on my elbow facing her, but not too close.

After finishing her sentence in the latest Harry Potter book, Karen set the book face-down on her pillow.

"What did I do now?" She clasped her hands and braced herself for another scolding. I'd been doing a lot of scolding.

"Nothing. I just need to tell you something about me. I know I've been really hard on you lately and grilling you about everything. I want to try to explain why I've been freaking out."

"Yeah, you've been a bit on the extreme side lately." She rolled her eyes and flipped over onto her back. I was getting used to the eye roll, and it didn't help me muster the courage to be vulnerable. I wanted to scold her for rolling her eyes again, but I knew this wasn't the time to fight. I was getting tired of fighting.

"I know." I took a deep breath and plunged in. "I've been a bit anxious because I remember what it was like for me when I was your age. I started smoking pot when I was twelve. By the time I was thirteen I was sneaking around behind my parents' backs and making all sorts of crazy choices. I know there are kids at your school who are doing the same things—probably even worse things now with all the new drugs out there. It scares me and I don't want you to make the same mistakes I did."

I stared at the Britney Spears poster on the wall wishing I had never let her buy that CD. I wanted her to stay innocent— forever—but I knew when she sang with Britney, "I'm not that innocent," to some degree it was true.

She didn't say anything, so I kept on with my nervous over-explanation.

"I know you're different than I was at your age. You have different parents, you're growing up in a much different environment, you have different friends and you'll make different choices. But I still worry, and I want to ask you to be patient with me. If I start freaking out and asking you about drugs and sex all the time, it's just because I'm remembering what I was doing at your age. Please understand, sometimes it's not about you. Sometimes it's about me and my own fears and hurts from *my* past coming to the surface. I want to trust you and believe you will make wise choices. I want to let you make some of your own mistakes and learn from them. But it's really hard."

"Okay, Mom, I understand." Karen rolled back over, picked up *Harry Potter and the Goblet of Fire* and lost herself in its pages.

I lingered a few moments longer, wondering if I should tell her more, but my real-life stories would never compete with the fantasy world of Hogwarts. I surrendered to her silence, wishing I could escape from my own painful past and keep her from falling into the same traps.

Facing Fears

I hoped Karen would understand and make better choices than I did, but there was nothing I could do to *make* her understand. No matter how hard I tried, I couldn't force her to make wise choices.

Part of me wanted to treat Karen like one of those perfect, long-stemmed red roses grown in the greenhouse for Valentine's Day. As parents we want our girls to be perfect flowers, so we create artificial environments, we shelter them, we breed out the thorns—no snarky behavior or critical thinking allowed. We want them to develop just to the point of budding and then cut them off and present them pure and perfect to the watching world, forever young, forever innocent, forever perfect.

Many youth groups use the image of a perfect rose to signify innocence and purity.[1] Some women have reported that such metaphors have harmed them.[2] Metaphors are powerful forces in shaping not only our worldview, but also our everyday interactions. What are some of the metaphors that have shaped how you view your daughter?

We would do well to remember that thorns develop on roses to protect them from climbing creatures who seek to devour them. While I desired to protect my daughter from the devouring dangers of drugs and sexual promiscuity, I needed to allow her to bloom and grow and develop her own thorns of protection. My job was to enrich the soil, not poison it. To expose her to the light, not hide her in the darkness of fear and shame.

Being vulnerable enough to tell Karen some of my fears helped show her that I am not perfect; I am a human in need of connection with God and others. I followed up with other flopping-down-on-her-bed conversations and tried to express my faith that she would make different choices than I had, that

I believed God was at work in her to help her make wise choices. I tried to assure her that I trusted she would learn from her own mistakes and that I would love her in and through all of them.

> **#facingthetalk:** Be honest with yourself about your fears and failures before talking with your girls about them. Vulnerability inspires courage. Examine your fears and find their source. Some of us need to face our own past failures. Others of us may have fears connected with our past successes. Whether we fear our girls will do the things we regret doing or won't do the things we celebrate from our past, we need to face those fears and allow God's love to overwhelm us with grace and peace.

Flipping a Switch, or the Great Disconnect

By the fourth day of early-morning text messages, I set an alarm to be sure I wouldn't miss her. At first I thought Kimberly, age twelve, was texting me all the time because she was excited to use her new phone. One day I didn't reply to her message and she called me later that evening and was upset. She explained that she really wanted to stay connected with me while I was out of town. It wasn't just about the new phone. We gave our girls their first phones when they were in seventh grade. Junior high seemed like a good milestone to celebrate this privilege and responsibility. It also provided a way for us to stay connected during a time when they were doing all they could do to disconnect from us as parents. This intense phase of disconnection is part of the differentiation process. During this phase, which often spans the age range of thirteen to eighteen, youth define themselves against their most intimate connections. In order to discover and become who they are created to be, they exaggerate the boundaries between themselves and those closest to them. This hadn't happened with Kimberly. Yet.

We texted or talked on the phone at least once a day while I was taking seminary classes in Portland that fall. And she was the first one to greet me with a hug after I returned home from my ten days away. I went to my bedroom early one night after returning from Portland. I had a stack of reading to do before posting online for my classes the next day.

"Mom, can I come and read with you?" Kimberly plopped down on her dad's side of the bed with Madeleine L'Engle's *A Wrinkle in Time* in her hands.

"Of course you can come read with me." I set my book on my lap and made room for her to snuggle up close.

We read peacefully until her eyes started falling shut between paragraphs. Her head fell toward the book, then she jerked awake seconds later and nudged me to get my attention.

"Mom, can I sleep in here with you?"

"You know you have to sleep in your own bed, sweetie. But you can stay here until your father comes to bed." I let her snuggle close until she fell asleep, cherishing every moment.

Whenever I would comment on her siblings' refusal to let me hug or touch them, Kimberly promised she would never stop snuggling with me. Ever. She often joined me as I read my seminary textbooks in bed in the evening, wanting to snuggle before getting in her own bed for the night. Change always adds a new level of anxiety to a family, even when it's good change. Career changes, new family members, siblings going off to college—all these are good changes, but stressors nonetheless. Since I was traveling more with work and school, I wanted to make myself available to Kimberly as much as possible when I was home. Her older sisters had already transitioned into teens who really didn't want to talk to me anymore anyway, so Kimberly's snuggling comforted me as much as it did her.

"Who's that sleeping in my bed?" Ken approached Kimberly like the Papa Bear in "Goldilocks and the Three Bears." But he's not a Papa Bear, so he reached down and tickled her awake.

"Time to go to bed, Kimbo." She grumbled and pushed his hand away as she rolled over, half-awake.

She practically fell off the bed and stumbled her way to her room with her eyes half-closed.

A few minutes later Ken climbed into bed. Like many other nights, he fell asleep minutes after turning his back on me.

Reflection. Ken and I were going through some rough times in our relationship at that point. We were in marriage counseling and working through our stuff, but it wasn't easy. I think the transition of our girls to adolescence was hard on him. He often took their opposition and disconnection personally. It's hard for parents not to feel rejected when our teens become more independent. And if we have any personal pain from past rejection or abandonment, this is often when it comes to the surface.

Often we worry about what our girls learn about sex and love from society, forgetting that family relationships have a much stronger influence on shaping their ideas about sex, love and marriage.

#selfcare: When girls transition into adolescence, parents need mentors or counselors to help them deal with anxiety and stress. Pay attention to how you're feeling as your girls transition into adolescence. Consider going to counseling if you find that you're becoming highly anxious, depressed or combative in your relationship with them. Remember, when they seem to be rejecting family values, they are not rejecting you. This intense phase of differentiation calls for love and acceptance of their differences.

I confess that I was tempted to get the majority of my affection needs met by Kimberly at this stage in my life. Many parents make the mistake of looking to their children to fulfill their relational needs when their marriages are lacking in some way. My counselor was wise enough to help me face that temptation head on. But while I was careful to seek God and seek help when my marriage was struggling, I also recognized that Kimberly's affection was a means of grace to me. While I was careful not to depend on her to meet my needs for affection, I was also careful not to push her away for fear of crossing some line. Sometimes we all need to experience Jesus with skin on. I am confident that Jesus was faithfully present in my relationship with Kimberly, helping me to tangibly experience God's love and compassion during a stressful time in our family.

Fortunately, things were on the mend with Ken and me when Kimberly's switch flipped six months later.

It was a wet February morning in Portland when I realized she hadn't called or texted me. It was day three of my ten-day trip to George Fox Evangelical Seminary that spring and I had texted her two mornings in a row without a response. So I called home after classes that night.

"Hi, Dear." The caller ID on Ken's cell phone told him it was me.

"Hi, Dear. How are you doing?" I closed the door to the guest room I was staying in at my friend's house in Portland.

"Fine." Ken has never been a big talker.

"How are the girls?"

"They're fine. They're all doing homework now."

"Wow. How'd you manage that?"

"I told them you'd be calling soon."

"You are so funny!"

"How are your classes?"

We talked awhile about my classes and his work and the details of the meals he'd prepared and the restaurants I'd visited.

"Do you want to talk to the girls?"

"Do they want to talk to me?"

I could hear him call to Kimberly as he held the phone away from his face. He called each one of their names and got the same response: *No thank you. I'm busy.*

"No, they're all busy." He affirmed what I already knew.

"That's okay. I'll be home soon enough. I'm sure they'll call me if they need something."

"Are you going to Skype in for family devotions on Sunday?"

"Yes, if we can get everything working this time."

"Okay, then. Love you and see you on Skype Sunday night."

"Love you too."

Reflection. After I started seminary, we discovered a good rhythm for family devotions and tried to stick with it even when I traveled. With the advances in video-chat technology, I was able to be virtually present for devotions even when I was out of town. This regular family gathering gave us an opportunity to connect consistently as a family so that when the girls were practicing their disconnecting, I didn't have to fear. I didn't feel the need to force them to talk with me on the phone. I knew we would connect in a few days. Having a planned time for family connection helps make room for periods of disconnection to be safe and healthy.

One of my favorite metaphors from one of our marriage counselors—one that applies to more than just marriage—is the idea that relationships with others are like an accordion. People in relationships are like the two wood boxes of an accordion. When kept apart from one another, they're merely two wooden boxes with reeds and grilles, buttons and keys. There is no music when the boxes are apart. When held together, they may appear to be close—to be as one—but there is no music flowing in the lack of space between them. With an accordion, it's the moving together and apart, separate and then close, that makes the music flow. So it is in relationships. It's the unique patterns played on the buttons and keys of individual lives moving in rhythm with one another that play the songs our hearts can hear.

Our weekly family devotional time provided the rhythm for the music of our family to flow as our girls learned to be separate from us while staying connected. We gathered each Sunday night to watch our favorite animated TV show together—*The Simpsons*. Afterward we would talk about a Bible passage we'd read that week and then pray together. When we knew we would be together on Sunday nights, Ken and I felt a little less anxious about the ways our girls were separating from us. We also tried to have family dinners together a few times each week. By the time our girls reached the age of twelve or thirteen, they spent the majority of their time apart from us—whether in school, in activities or in seclusion in their rooms. So family dinners and family devotions became even more important.

#facingthetalk: Puberty is about more than hormones; it's about identity development and healthy differentiation into adulthood. Recognize and talk about how things are changing for the whole family as each girl transitions into puberty. Talk about the changes in the social dynamics of the family. Establish new ways of connecting that affirm their need for privacy and personal space. Communicate your desire to stay connected even when they push back or reject you in one way or another. Accept their need to be separate more often, but establish regular routines for connection and togetherness. Be careful about overemphasizing hormones or periods during this transitional time. Many things are changing for them physically, socially, psychologically, emotionally and intellectually. Their desire for privacy and need for separateness is not always hormonal.

Is It Hormones?

"Don't touch me!" Karen snarled. If looks could kill, I would be dead a thousand times over.

I knew this day would come; I just didn't know it would come so soon. The first time it happened, thirteen-year-old Karen had just discovered the band Superchick and kept asking me to push replay on the song "We Live." I loved the lyrics and the music, so I gladly complied. There are some times when a mom benefits from her daughter's obsessions. This was one of them. It also opened the door for one of those blessed and prized teachable moments.

The song is a story about losing loved ones to cancer, an accident or another unexpected event. After pushing replay for the third time, I paused the Volvo's CD player in the middle of the song and asked Karen straight up whether she understood the lyrics. Then, without taking my eyes off the road for longer than a brief second, I shot her my "I really mean this" look—the one that's supposed to inspire life, not death.

"This is why I won't stop hugging you," I said. "And this is why you need to let me. We just never know which day will be our last."

I kept my focus on the road, trying not to let the tears sneak through and choke out my words. After that day in the car, Karen rarely responded with such anger to my requests to touch her or hug her.

Reflection. I wish such teachable moments on every parent. This happened in the spring of seventh grade for Karen, and not long after that day she came up to me at church on Mother's Day and gave me a big, long hug—in public, no less! In front of her friends, in front of her friends' parents, in front of her

Sunday school teachers. This time I couldn't stop the words from catching in my throat; I couldn't swallow the tears. I knew she remembered the song. I knew she still loved me no matter how many other days she pushed me away or called me names or told me she hated me. That moment made it all clear—those other things were true for a moment, but they were fleeting. This bond would last.

As you prepare to take your daughter on a second getaway after the switch has already flipped and she has become oppositional, doesn't want to talk about it, rejects your affectionate overtures and flinches every time you try to touch her, don't worry. And don't take it personally. I've heard it happens even to the best of parents.

> **#facingthetalk:** Talk honestly about the need to stay connected through affectionate physical touch with family. Healthy touch heals. Celebrate the moments of connection, even if they're brief and fleeting. Invite them to participate in making the choice of when and how to embrace. It's hard to force affectionate touch. Something about forcing it makes it feel less affectionate. Instead of requiring them to hug or kiss whenever you want to, ask permission.

Late Bloomers and PMS

"Kimberly has boobies!" eighteen-year-old Karen announced to Nana as Kimberly came down the stairs.

"Karen, that was rude!" Kimberly gave my mom—AKA Nana—a big hug while giving Karen the death stare.

"Oh my gosh, you have grown up so much! You are developing into quite a lovely young lady," Nana said, looking around to see if Papa, my stepdad, had come inside with the luggage. Nope, no men in the room. So she went on to probe into more intimate girly matters.

"Have you started your period?" Nana inquired in a more hushed tone than Karen's broadcast announcement about Kimberly's boobies.

"No, Nana, I'm only twelve."

"I know, but you look so grown up. You're not my little Kimmy anymore." Nana pulled her close for a longer-than-is-comfortable-for-a-preteen hug.

"Where are Kelly and Katie?" Nana sat down at the green granite kitchen counter.

"They're probably in their rooms reading. Kim, will you go tell Kelly and Katie that Nana and Papa are here?" Papa had settled in the daddy chair in the family room, tired and ready for a nap after the long drive.

"Has Kelly started her period yet?" Nana asked. Kelly was fourteen at the time.

"No, not yet," Karen answered as her Nana played with her long red curls. "Wouldn't it be crazy if Kimberly started before Kelly?"

"It's totally possible at the rate Kimberly's developing," I said. I heard Kelly yell at Kimberly to leave her alone. Kelly hated to be roused from her afternoon naps.

"It's amazing how each daughter is so different," I said. "But I sure hope Kelly starts her period soon. It seems like she's been PMS-ing for over a year now." I sat down on a barstool next to my mom and began to reminisce with her.

Reflection. Kelly was a bit of a late bloomer. She didn't start walking until she was eighteen months old, and she wasn't an early talker like her two older sisters. We attributed much of this to the fact that her sisters did everything for her and interpreted her needs to us so she didn't have to talk. As a baby she insisted on being held whenever we were away from home.

She was clingy as a toddler—even up until first grade. I remember dragging her into school one day and leaving her crying with her first grade teacher. I spent the next ten minutes in the nurse's office making sure I was doing the right thing. I think it was more traumatic for me than for her. Now, at seventeen years old, she barely remembers the incident. But her tears are seared onto my memory.

You can imagine how dramatic it was for Ken and me when Kelly's switch flipped. The little girl who always wanted to sit as close to me as possible on the couch, who climbed onto her daddy's lap at the most awkward times and inconvenient places, was suddenly refusing to let us touch her and vehemently pushing us away when we got too close. I used to think her clinginess was a birth order thing, but this radical switch made me reconsider everything. I'm sure birth order played some part in her personality development, but my guess is that her extremes in behavior were more related to her natural temperament than anything else. Learning to understand my girls' personality types, learning styles and unique passions has helped me treat each one with respect and dignity.

While each girl is unique and transitioned into puberty differently, one thing remained the same—they did transition. The switch always flipped.

Most of us mark the end of this transition time by the onset of menses, and this was the marker Ken and I used as well. We had distinct terms we used for the girls for different stages of development marked by significant events. Here were our markers:

- Baby: prewalking
- Little girl: walking but still in diapers

- Big girl: walking and potty trained—they remain a big girl for a long time!
- Young woman/young lady: after onset of menses
- Woman: after age 18

I always made a big deal about my girls starting their period. It embarrassed them, but I did it anyway. Lisa McMinn in *Sexuality and Holy Longing* reminds us of how important it is to celebrate this transition and help our girls develop healthy positive attitudes about this special bodily function: "The collective shame and hate of menstruation that women share has emerged partly out of a long-running history of considering femaleness inferior to maleness. Many societies considered female sexuality not only as being dangerous, but as causing women to be frail, irrational, and illogical."[3] She goes on to encourage menstruation rituals that impart blessing and help girls think redemptively about their embodied sexuality.

McMinn suggests that teaching our girls a healthy view of their bodies by celebrating the onset of menses helps them start to understand that menstruation is about more than having babies. Our bodies are a beautiful mix of mystery and mastery. While we are responsible to learn how to take care of our bodies, how to exercise self-control, how to use our bodies to accomplish things in the world, and how to interact with others in our bodies, there are still many things about our bodies that are out of our control and beyond our comprehension. McMinn writes, "Women inhabit physical bodies that menstruate every month, and their personhood cannot be separated from their bodies. Attending to a cycle that is fundamental to women's physical nature opens the door for potential insight and unexpected blessing."[4]

As girls transition into puberty, they become increasingly

self-conscious and it's often hard to celebrate. But we did it anyway. While the first mother-daughter getaway was a celebration of God's good intention for creation and sex, the second getaway was a chance to celebrate the goodness of femaleness—including menstruation. A good time to schedule this second getaway is after your daughter starts menstruating. And that can be challenging since the timing of the onset of menses is so unpredictable. Almost as unpredictable as the mood changes during this time of transition.

PMS, or premenstrual syndrome, is a real thing, but not everyone has it. PMS is a vague and general term for an assortment of symptoms occurring prior to menses, but mostly it's associated with negative moods, emotional sensitivity and irritability.

Too often we use PMS as an excuse for bad behavior or overlook other problems by labeling all mood swings, sensitivity and negative emotions as PMS. One study shows that women who reported PMS symptoms had the same level of hormones as other women who reported no symptoms. The conclusion of the study was that it's not the levels of hormones that cause the PMS symptoms, but rather a sensitivity to the fluctuation of hormone levels and variation in pain sensitivity levels.

At this stage of development, it's important to remember that not all emotional changes are related to reproductive function. There are many other factors influencing mood and sensitivity, including stress, diet, relationships and sleep patterns, that should be considered. Labeling all moodiness as PMS reinforces negative stereotypes about menstruation and continues the culture of shame and hate surrounding menstruation.

Too often women are shamed for expressing their complex emotions, labeled crazy and expected to get their emotions under control. Hormonal shifts do not cause emotions, but certain hormones can intensify feelings. Be careful not to dismiss your daughter's feelings, especially the overwhelming feelings that such intensity might cause. Recognize that some feelings may be new and scary, such as feeling sad and depressed when rejected by a friend or feeling sexual attraction for the first time.

> **#facingthetalk:** Many changes happen during puberty, not just reproductive changes. Not all moodiness, anxiety or irritability is hormonal. Pay attention to sadness, anxiety and other emotional changes and treat them as possible opportunities to connect with your daughter in meaningful ways. Rejoice with her over new crushes and weep with her over new losses. Be careful about using PMS as a way of dismissing the complex emotions that arise during this time of transition. Don't label all moodiness, anxiety or irritability as PMS or related to reproductive hormones.

Changes in Preteen Years

From ages nine to thirteen, sexual development is very active. Preteens continue to be curious about sexuality, usually because they are more aware of the impending changes to their bodies, but also because they are exposed to increasing numbers of sexual messages in the media. Some girls start having periods and their breasts begin to develop. Boys' voices change, and they start to grow pubic hair. These changes can make young people feel uncomfortable, embarrassed and suddenly very private.

This stage of individuation also begins a period of extreme distance and separation from the family system. In a child's quest to understand and define who she is, these years mark a transition into a period of defining who she is not, over and against those closest to her.

During these times of rapid change and intense individuation, children often have questions about the physical changes their bodies are going through. It can be hard for adults to discuss these things. Girls start looking grown-up, but they're still children. Some girls start feeling embarrassed more easily. But it's important both for children and adults to talk about sexuality and the changes our girls are experiencing. Here are some characteristics of this time of change:

- Most girls start to develop breasts and have their first period by age thirteen.

- Some girls become worried and anxious if their physical development is more or less advanced than their peers.

- Body image becomes increasingly important and peer opinion is valued over family standards.

- Preteens often develop intense admiration for same-sex adults. They may transition from having an intense and strong relationship with the same-sex parent to having a distant and oppositional relationship, shifting their intensity to other adult role models.

- Girls may begin having crushes, become more interested in romantic relationships and desire to have a boyfriend.

- For some, masturbation is a response to new urges or intensifies for those who have masturbated as a comfort when younger. For others, the desire to masturbate never crosses their mind or body. Masturbation is more common for developing boys, but is not unheard of for developing girls.

- Curiosity about adult bodies, including trying to see people naked or undressing, may increase or intensify. Girls may become more interested in TV, movies, websites and magazines with sexual content.

- Only 15 percent of girls are exposed to porn by age thirteen.

In recent studies, the majority of young girls have reported that they do not want to view pornographic images and have not sought them out. But with increasing access to porn on the Internet and increased curiosity, the risk of exposure is rising.

- Differences between male and female become more noticeable and distinct. Girl culture and boy culture begin to draw girls and boys into separate social spheres. They may drop childhood friends of the opposite sex during this time.

Reflection. I often found myself focused on and worried about my daughters and their development, forgetting that I was developing too. The ways I interacted with my oldest daughter and my younger daughters around these topics changed over time. It's helpful for us parents to remember that we are in process as much as our daughters are. We can model healthy growth for them by being willing to adapt and change with them.

Developmental process doesn't stop when we hit adulthood. While it seems like some of the biggest shifts happen between the ages of thirteen and seventeen, we can also experience major shifts between the ages of thirty and forty. As the age of first marriage is rising to an average of twenty-seven years old and many women are having children later as well, it's not uncommon for mothers to be transitioning through menopause at the same time as their daughters are transitioning through puberty. Pay attention to the shifts happening in your own life and how those might affect your family system.

#selfcare: Adolescents aren't the only ones who go through major transitions in life. Seek out trusted advisers to talk to about your own transitions.

When Ken and I first went through counseling at our church, we were told that many adults seek help with issues from their childhood when they're in their thirties. I have heard this from other counselors and psychologists as well. One theory is that people in their thirties have reached a certain emotional maturity, so they're able to process their past in productive ways. Another theory is that the pressures of life become significant enough during midlife that people are motivated to seek help. For me, it was the pressures of having four daughters that prompted me to seek counsel. The next chapter recalls some issues from my past that surfaced as I worked with counselors and mentors over the years.

These personal narratives give context to why I have approached talking with my daughters about sex in the ways I describe in this book. Some of these connections I have made in retrospect; others were experienced in the midst of conversations with my girls. I hope that reading my stories will help you make connections with your own past—connections that will help you recognize any fear and shame that arise as you talk with your own girls.

Back Story

When I trapped Karen in the car on my first attempt to talk with her about sex, I had no idea how significant that trip would be in dealing with trauma from my past. Looking back, I realize that visiting my dad triggered fear and anxiety in me that probably spilled over onto Karen.

We had visited my dad at Sunrise of Decatur, the nursing home where he was being cared for. We were afraid the place would smell terrible. But we were pleasantly surprised. As we approached the palatial facility, we were struck by the two Rapunzel-like towers that emerged at the end of each wing. I wondered if my dad felt trapped in there.

The lobby was spotless, just like the home my dad had lived in for over thirty years. We signed the guest book and waited to be granted permission to enter the fortress of care. The Alzheimer's memory care unit was secured with a code to open doors and operate elevators that only staff and registered guests were given. My dad was locked in for his own safety.

It seemed ironic that my sister and I had spent years locking ourselves in our room at night to keep ourselves safe from our dad, and now he was the one locked up to keep him safe from himself. He had stopped hurting us years ago, but the fear and shame lived on.

I hadn't yet arrived at a state of feeling safe. Even after years of counseling—with my sister, with my husband and on my own—I still experienced high levels of anxiety. My anxiety was often expressed in attempts to control others' emotions. I felt trapped. Imprisoned by fear. One of my biggest anxieties was that I would turn out like my dad and harm my kids. No matter how far away he lived or how infrequently I saw him, I could never escape his presence in my life. He was my dad. I didn't choose him to be my dad. And I certainly didn't choose to grow up in a family that perpetuated cycles of abuse handed down from generation to generation. But I had to deal with those realities whether I liked it or not.

I'm sure it was the sense of feeling trapped in an abusive family system that motivated me to talk to my girls about sex. Like Rapunzel, I longed for a means of escape. I hoped that talking to them about God's good plan for sex would help protect them from experiencing the fear and shame I had grown up with. But unlike Rapunzel, I didn't live in a fairy-tale world of magical healing or fanciful happily-ever-afters.

On top of that, after our last daughter, Kimberly, was born, I reached my pressure point. I've heard that God often allows circumstances in our lives to put just the right amount of pressure on us to reveal what's really in our hearts. And what was in my heart was not pretty. I'll never forget the day I first realized I was becoming like my dad.

Meatloaf and Madness

The meatloaf was in the oven and I was preparing homemade

macaroni and cheese on the stove. The pot of water had just started boiling as I added the cheese to my roux. As I dumped the noodles into the boiling water, I heard Kelly begin to whine and cry. Ken and the girls were in the family room, just a split level below the kitchen with a half-wall in between. I was already stressed out by the cooking—I can never get the timing right so the food is all ready at the same time—and Kelly's crying ramped my stress level up a notch.

I started slicing the cheddar cheese for the sauce, trusting that Ken would take care of Kelly. But the whining and crying didn't stop. Instead it escalated into one of her infamous fits. *What is going on down there? What is she crying about? Why doesn't he take care of it?*

I tossed the cheddar into the sauce and stirred the noodles so they wouldn't boil over before I made a break for the family room. I stood at the top of the steps to survey the scene.

Karen was on the far side of the room playing with Kimberly on the baby blanket, while Katie zoom-zoomed with the cars in her toy garage. Ken was sitting in his favorite recliner reading the paper. Kelly was just a few feet away pitching her fit.

"Ken! Why don't you pick her up? She obviously needs something!"

Ken kept reading the article he was in the middle of as I descended the stairs.

"She'll be fine," he said after he looked up from the paper a few moments later.

Those moments felt like forever.

I picked Kelly up, feeling furious. The rage in my heart was way out of proportion to what the situation warranted, but I didn't know that. All I knew was that I was very angry. Not with Kelly—kids just pitch a fit sometimes. I was angry that

Ken was sitting there doing nothing. Parents aren't supposed to do that.

"I need you to take her and take care of this," I told him. "I'm trying to get dinner prepared and the table set and I'm already stressed as it is. I don't need to hear her pitching a fit while I'm trying to concentrate on getting dinner ready!"

My mean, mad mom voice didn't move him. He just sat there staring at me.

"How can you sit there and do nothing? Don't you care about her? Don't you care about me? I need you to take care of this *now*!"

And then it happened.

I threw Kelly across the room.

She landed in a pile of blankets unharmed. But the damage done in that moment cannot be measured in numbers of broken bones.

I had just abused my own daughter.

Something I vowed I would never do.

I waited for Ken to rescue me. I wanted him to pick Kelly up and tell me I was a horrible mom. I wanted him to insist that I get out of the house and see a therapist immediately. But he didn't do anything. He just sat there—unconsciously paralyzed by emotions from his own childhood.

The timer went off and I retreated to the kitchen to finish preparing dinner. The noodles had boiled over and the meatloaf was nearly burned. I took the overcooked meatloaf out of the oven, stirred the cheese sauce and drained the noodles.

"Do you need help with dinner?" Ken stood at the threshold to the kitchen.

I could hardly think straight to figure out what to do next, let alone give him instructions on how to help me.

"Yes, I could use help! You could help by taking care of the kids while I finish getting everything ready. Dinner will be on the table in five minutes."

The next day I called the counseling ministry at our church and scheduled an appointment for Ken and me. I couldn't wait any longer for him to rescue me. I needed help right away. I needed to stop the cycle of abuse before I did more of what I had vowed I would never do—abuse my children, and my husband.

We went to counseling at church together for six weeks. In that period it became apparent that many of our problems stemmed from our childhood family systems. I was ready to deal with my past, but I needed more than six weeks of relationship advice to heal the deep wounds in my heart. I ended up going to a professional counselor who helped me work through many of my issues from childhood trauma and abuse. She helped me take steps to begin to break the cycle of abuse.

> **#selfcare:** If you have experienced abuse or trauma in your past, seek professional help. Be kind to yourself and choose healing. Nobody else is going to choose it for you.

During my time in counseling, we explored themes of abandonment and rejection that were likely roots of my fear and shame, which inspired me to be controlling and hypervigilant in my relationship with my husband and children. Fear and shame don't always manifest this way, but in my case they did. While this book is not a marriage guide, there is without a doubt a connection between what we experience in our most intimate relationships and how we talk about sex and intimacy with our girls.

As my oldest daughter transitioned into a teen, my fear and hypervigilance increased significantly, though I didn't make the connection at the time. One of the memories of rejection that plagued me often was when my best friend's boyfriend made a pass at me in junior high.

My Best Friend's Boyfriend

I loved the way I felt in that moment—his touch set my whole body aflame. But I pushed him away.

"Jerry! Stop! What are you doing? Kel is going to be so mad at you."

"I won't tell if you don't." He tried tickling my ribs but I squirmed away and slammed through the metal door into the hallway.

He ran beside me as we passed my friend Megan running the opposite direction. A few wordless strides later, he ran on ahead and left me breathless. What the hell was that? I was conflicted.

That kiss felt good, but I feel bad. Why did he kiss me when he's dating my friend Kel? Should I tell Kel or keep it a secret? What if he tries it again? Why would he do that to Kel? Oh my, he's so gorgeous and such a good kisser. Can I catch up with him and kiss him again?

Jerry wasn't the first boy I kissed. And he wasn't the first boy who kissed me while choosing to love another. Something similar had happened to me in sixth grade, and it broke my heart, making me feel like I wasn't quite good enough. I was someone to make out with secretly but not someone to go public with.

Jerry's actions reinforced those feelings. However, I let him carry on. My body longed for his touch, but each time he snuck a kiss behind Kel's back, I felt increasingly dirty and unlovable. I don't know why I kept letting him do it. Perhaps I thought a secret love was better than no love at all.

Reflection. This is just one of the memories that haunted me and yet inspired me to talk to my girls about sex. I didn't feel comfortable telling them the true stories—I couldn't share those memories with them. But could I protect them from the heartache and rejection? Could I spare them from the feelings of fear and shame? The memories didn't often surface in vivid detail, but they seeped into my semiconsciousness, affecting the choices I made as a parent. On some days my desperation was palpable. I wanted my girls to feel loved and accepted more than I did at their age. Unfortunately, no matter how hard I tried, I couldn't control their social world. I couldn't even control their family system!

A family system is a complex system of interdependent, unpredictable people. I only have control over one part of it—myself. As I find healing and freedom from fear and shame, I am learning to give up worrying about things I have no control over. This healing has had a positive impact on those closest to me. But my years of struggle had impact as well.

Much of my fear was connected to feelings of rejection and abandonment. While those feelings also inspired shame, some of the deepest shame I felt was over my decision to have sex at age sixteen.

Rumors and Reputations

The rumor spread like wildfire.

At least that's how it felt to me.

"Did you hear what Johnny said about you?" Mandy asked me between classes.

"No, I haven't talked to him since we made out in the back of the bus at the basketball game last Friday. What did he say?" I slammed my locker shut as I turned to walk to class with Mandy.

"I overheard him talking to Mark about how easy you were and how much you wanted him. He was making a really big deal

about it." Mandy grabbed my arm so she wouldn't lose me as we
wove through the sea of students in the hall.

"But we didn't even do it! All we did was kiss and he felt me
up—that's all!" My heart started to race as I spotted Johnny
coming down the hall toward us. I looked his way to say hi.

He didn't even see me.

"Mandy, did you see that? He ignored me. As if I didn't even
exist. He's talking about me behind my back and won't even say
hi to my face in the hall! What a jerk. I can't believe I made out
with him. I'm so stupid." I clutched Mandy's hand, which was
still clasped around my arm, to steady myself. I wanted to run
away and hide. But we had to go to math class.

It didn't take long before I was getting asked for sexual favors by
random guys at almost every party I attended. The assumption was
that I was not a virgin and enjoyed having sex for the fun of it.

The problem was, it wasn't true.

At least not all of it. Like many young teenage women, I was
passionate about kissing young teenage men. Making out at
sporting events or parties got my heart racing and juices flowing
for sure. Guys aren't the only ones who get horny. The problem
is, it's seen as natural for high school guys; when gals get horny,
they're viewed in a negative light.

A few weeks later I was making out with my friend's brother
Brady. He was a couple of years older than I was and really attractive. I liked him more than he liked me, so we weren't officially dating—more like what some might call "friends with
benefits" nowadays.

"Brady, I really want to have sex with you," I confessed as
things were heating up between us.

"But you're a virgin, right?" The rumor hadn't made it to Brady
yet.

"Yes, but everybody thinks I've had sex and my friends tell me it's great. I've even heard that you're great in bed. If I'm going to have a reputation for having already had sex, I may as well enjoy it!" I grabbed his bare chest as I spilled my guts. Then I kissed him again.

One thing I loved about Brady: I could always be honest and straightforward with him. And we definitely had chemistry.

Our bodies moved in synchrony as I tried to persuade him.

But he stopped me and refused.

"You don't want me to be your first. Really. You should fall in love and it should be special. It should be with someone who really cares about you—I mean, you know I care about you, but not in that way. Your first time should be with someone who's committed to you and wants to make lasting memories with you. I'm just a guy who likes to play around. I don't want to be your first. You deserve better." He stroked my cheek gently, but nothing could soften the blow of rejection.

Tears started welling up in my eyes.

He wiped away one that escaped.

I fell asleep with my head on his shoulder for a while. Then he took me home.

The next day I woke up even more determined to live up to my new reputation. I wanted to follow Brady's advice to wait until I fell in love, but true love didn't seem to be close on any of my horizons.

A few months later I found a guy who was willing to be my first. We met on our senior class trip. I won't narrate the details for you, but one thing is for sure—it wasn't true love. He was a foreign exchange student and our "lovemaking" was merely a weekend fling.

Reflection. When I think about my junior high and high

school romances, I still experience lingering feelings of shame and regret. But instead of focusing on the negative emotions from my past, I choose to look for healing and grace.

Even though I felt rejected and abandoned, I know I am loved and accepted by God.

Even though I chose to have sex for the first time with someone I didn't really love, I believe I am loved and accepted by God.

I have to keep reminding myself of these things because fear and shame are compelling emotional forces that stealthily invade our everyday lives.

Much of what I chose to do on my first How-To getaway with Karen was motivated by fear.

A few years later, much of what I did on her How-Not-To getaway was driven by shame.

6

The How-Not-To Sex Talk

The statistics show that (almost) everyone is doing it before they get married—even Christians.[1] I remind myself that statistics are a description of past behavior, not a prediction of the future. I tell myself that just because I had sex at age sixteen, that doesn't mean my daughters will. While some speculate about why young Christians aren't waiting anymore, I look for the reasons why some *are* waiting.[2] I hope my girls will make better choices than I did. Isn't that what most parents want?

If I could just spare her that pain—the pain of feeling dirty and unlovable after having casual sex, I thought. If I could just make sure she knows she's special, valuable and worthy of love.

I didn't know for certain whether a purity talk and signing a purity pledge would protect Karen from the shame I had experienced or help her feel special, but I hoped it would make some kind of difference. I searched the local Christian bookstores and looked online and finally found a program called Passport2Purity. Before Karen's thirteenth birthday, I invited her best friend and her mom to do a Passport2Purity weekend together. We hoped our daughters might be a little more receptive to our instruction if we had someone else to back us up.

How-Not-To Sex Talk No. 1

Glue, construction paper, puzzles, balloons—we gathered the supplies listed in the Passport2Purity parent guide and embarked on my first How-Not-To weekend getaway. My first attempt to talk with Karen about sex on the How-To getaway had felt like a failure. This time I was going to be prepared and do it right. I'd heard stories from some older Christians who raised their kids up right—their kids had waited until marriage to have sex and everything was perfect. That was the kind of Christian parent I wanted to be—the kind who did things the right way.

I received the Passport2Purity curriculum in the mail. It was a small box containing a set of CDs, a parent guide and a student guide; the student guide included a purity pledge card dressed up like a passport. It felt like it would grant me access to the ideal Christian future I imagined.

I invited my friend DeBorah and her daughter Kelsea to join us on the getaway. Kelsea and Karen had been friends since fourth grade and DeBorah had become an encouraging friend and prayer partner. Everything we needed for our weekend getaway was provided in the little box except for the supplies for the object lessons and the destination for our getaway. For our destination we picked Harrison Hot Springs Resort.

It was about a three-hour drive from Seattle to the resort, so we started listening to the CDs on the way in the car. There was something about having a captive audience that made it easier.

At the end of one of the sessions we were instructed to do the water balloon activity.

"Where are we going to fill up the balloons?" Karen asked.

"We can do it when we stop for lunch," DeBorah suggested.

We read through the instructions in the parent guide. The activity required the girls to each fill up a water balloon and use a pin to poke holes in it.

"You mean, like, fill it up in a public bathroom? Gross!" Kelsea chimed in.

We stopped at an A&W for lunch. After I finished my root beer float, I got the supplies out of the back of the car and went to the bathroom to fill up the balloons. Back outside, I handed the balloons to Karen and Kelsea, then flipped open the parent guide to the right page.

"Imagine the water inside the balloon is your sexual purity and innocence. It's all you have," I read from the guide. "Now, imagine your first kiss."

DeBorah pierced Kelsea's balloon with a pin to let just a drop of water out. Karen's balloon didn't pierce easily, but eventually we made a tiny hole.

"Now imagine another boy comes along and wants a kiss or maybe just a little more than a kiss." We pierced the balloons a few more times and they started dripping.

"Let's say you fall in love and decide that it's okay to give even more of your purity and innocence away." We pierced the balloons again until streams of water started flowing out onto the pavement.

"Oh no; they're really leaking fast!" Karen cried. Just then her balloon burst open.

Kelsea jumped back to avoid getting splashed and dropped her balloon onto the hot pavement with yet another splash.

"Well, that didn't work out as planned." Karen began to snicker.

We all burst out giggling. It was hard to finish reading the guided dialogue about losing one of the most precious gifts one can give another human being when we were standing in a fast-food parking lot with shreds of balloon all around us.

Afterward, I felt a bit deflated myself. While I enjoyed the levity, I worried that it would minimize the gravity of the illustration. I tried not to let my frustration show as we got back into the car to finish our drive to the resort. We decided to take a break from listening so we could do the activities in a more manageable setting.

We arrived at the resort and checked in at the front desk. It was teatime in the lobby, and there were cookies and little sandwiches available to snack on before we went to our room. Our room in the newly updated wing of the hotel had a stunning view of the surrounding mountains. The beds were covered with down comforters and the room smelled like new carpet.

"Can we go down to the pool?" Karen kicked off her shoes and ran to the bathroom to change into her bathing suit.

"Yeah, I'm ready to get out and do something. That was a long car ride." Kelsea patiently waited her turn to use the bathroom and change.

"Sure, go have fun at the pool. We'll join you in a bit." DeBorah picked the bed closest to the window for us to share. We knew Karen and Kelsea wouldn't want to sleep with their moms.

"Don't forget these." I handed robes to the girls. "They're provided by the hotel so you can cover up while walking through the halls to the pool. Towels are on a counter out by the pool. See you in a few minutes. We have some planning to do before we join you."

I walked over to the grocery bag full of supplies on the table and began to unpack the glue, construction paper and puzzles.

After unpacking and setting up the supplies, we headed out to soak in the pure mineral water with Karen and Kelsea. We soaked and swam, enjoying the time of relaxation after our long drive. When we returned to our room, we listened to the next session on the CD.

Reflection. The Passport2Purity curriculum was good, but after going through it a few times, I started to have some reservations. I found myself using it less and less with each daughter. By the time it was my youngest daughter Kimberly's turn, I switched to *The Purity Code* book and CD. You may find another curriculum that works well for you. Be sure to read the reviews and think about the metaphors presented before using any program. Metaphors have a powerful, world-shaping influence on our thinking. I provide my reviews of some available resources in appendix A, but ask other trusted advisers for their recommendations as well.

The way ideas are presented in any given curriculum can have unintended consequences. Some young women have reported feeling deep shame as a result of images such as the leaky balloon. But the curriculum is not the most important part of these getaways—it's continuing the conversation and making things that are often undiscussable between parents and children discussable. Fortunately, I feel like it's worked for me. I continue to have conversations with my girls about sex and purity to this day.

While sex and intimacy are private matters meant to consist of special moments between two people, keeping things secret and hidden promotes a sense of shame and fear. Using a curriculum helped me organize my thinking and talking. And the curriculum touched on subjects I may not have thought to talk about. Writing this book has also opened up the door for continuing conversations, but you don't have to be a writer to keep the dialogue going. Take pictures or videos of your getaway experiences and go back and watch them as your girls get older. Reminiscing together and thinking about what you might do differently as you grow and change helps them understand that maturity is an ongoing process, even for parents.

The Passport2Purity curriculum also helped me communicate a Christian standard of purity that was somewhat foreign to me. I have been exposed to a variety of views on sexuality—from the free love mentality of growing up in Woodstock, New York, to the conservative Christian view of "kissing dating goodbye" and waiting until marriage even to kiss. When I planned my first How-Not-To getaway, I wasn't exactly sure where I would land on the spectrum with my girls, but I was pretty sure it wouldn't be on the free love and sex end.

Much of my energy that weekend with Karen and our friends was spent getting supplies in order and making sure we stuck to our schedule. We would listen to a lesson, do an activity and guided discussion, then take a break to go in the pools, have a meal or go exploring. There wasn't much spontaneity to the weekend. To be honest, there wasn't much spontaneity in my life at all at that time. I wasn't ready to face the unknown of adolescence with my daughter, so I worked very hard to make life predictable.

I hoped that going through Passport2Purity and signing a purity pledge would convince Karen to wait until she was deeply loved and married to have sex. I hoped the curriculum would help me provide her a safe passage into adulthood. I imagined that keeping her purity intact would spare Karen the pain of rejection that I had felt when I had casual sex.

One of the things I appreciated about the curriculum when

I first bought it was the very specific instructions—I felt like I
needed someone to tell me what to do. I didn't trust myself to
know how to talk with my daughter about purity since I had
given up my virginity at such a young age. Instead, I let a curriculum do the talking for me.

Looking back, though, I find it hard to believe we told our
girls that they contained a source of purity that could be so
easily lost. As if purity were something they were born with, like
the hymen covering the vagina. Aren't such purity codes main-
tained only in societies where women and children are considered property? Surely the God of second chances, the compassionate God who offered the woman at the well access to
springs of living water, didn't expect my daughter to keep and
maintain her purity on her own.

The idea that purity equals virginity is being challenged today.
Jessica Valenti in *The Purity Myth* opens her book by saying, "It's
time to teach our daughters that their ability to be good people
depends on their *being good people*, not on whether or not they're
sexually active."[3] I would add that as Christians we want to
teach our daughters that their ability to be good people depends
on their connection to the source of all goodness—God.

Perhaps we need to teach our girls that purity is more like the
mineral hot springs we were swimming in. Purity is not something they need to keep safe inside a water balloon to give as a
gift to their future spouse. Purity is something they can enter
into at any time in their life. Whenever they enter into the life-
giving love of God, their hearts will be purified over and over
again by their faith.

You might worry that such ideas will give our girls license to
have sex whenever they want, and to some degree you would be
right. That's part of what being human is all about. God created

us with the freedom to choose our source of life. And when we choose to look for life in places other than the heart of God, we are covered by grace. It's God's boundless mercy and endless grace that lead us closer to God's heart—not a set of purity codes, not the law.

Whether we like it or not, our girls will choose when they want to have sex. We can influence how and why they make that choice, but we cannot make it for them. No matter how much we want to protect them, no matter how their choices will affect us, no matter how we want to believe they are a pure and innocent gift to be saved and given to another intact, we must remember that they are human beings with the capacity to act and make choices on their own. They are not our possessions. They belong to God, and we are God's stewards.

As stewards, we are responsible to train our girls and guide their choices. When they're little, we make many choices for them, but as they get older we must help them understand the freedom God grants all humans. By asking our daughters to sign a purity pledge before they're old enough to make such significant choices on their own, in one sense we're trying to make that choice for them. We are asking them to take a vow that may cause more harm than good.[4]

Jesus warns us about making vows in Matthew 5:33-37. In verse 37 he says, "All you need to say is simply 'Yes' or 'No'; anything beyond this comes from the evil one." When we ask our daughters to sign a purity pledge, we are not presenting them with a choice. We can help prepare them for the decision of saying yes or no when the choice of having sex is before them, but having them make a vow has not proved to be the best way to do that. Instead, making and breaking vows can lead to shame. And shame is our enemy.

Jesus promised that whoever believed in him would never be ashamed. It's not God's grace that leads to shame; it's the law. Whoever believes in the law, whoever depends on purity codes as a source of life, will likely find themselves immersed in shame. As for me, I prefer to immerse myself in God's abundant springs of grace-filled living water.

> **#facingthetalk:** Teach good decision making and trust your girls to make wise choices. Don't require them to make vows that lead to shame if broken.
>
> Talk to your girls about the true source of purity and what it means to have the freedom to choose when and with whom they have sex. We can't make this choice for them, no matter how much we want to. Religious sexual shame is a disease of the mind—and it's prudent to avoid psychological diseases as well as physical diseases.

Each of my daughters is unique, and I tried to tailor each experience to that girl's personality and interests. While I used a packaged curriculum, there was nothing packaged about the getaways. My goal, however, remained the same for each one— to create a strong bond and facilitate open and ongoing conversations about sex.

How-Not-To Sex Talk No. 2

Since Katie was an avid reader, devouring Harry Potter and other long books within a day or two, I decided to take her to Portland and Powell's City of Books for her getaway when she was thirteen. We took the train and the bus to our destination. We arrived at our hotel late in the afternoon, checked into our room for the weekend and listened to a couple of sessions.

We stayed at McMenamin's Kennedy School, a once-condemned elementary school that was saved by the devotion of former students and renovated to become a unique and fun lodging, dining and meeting experience. It was the perfect place to do arts and crafts.

"Katie, will you get the glue and construction paper out of the bag?" I asked. "We're going to start one of the activities before we go to dinner. After dinner we can watch the movie I brought."

I had seen the movie *Saved!* with the young adults at our local church and decided to watch it with Katie as one of our evening activities. It's a satirical teen comedy about a girl attending a Christian high school who becomes pregnant when she decides to have sex to "save" her boyfriend from being gay. She finds herself ostracized and demonized when all her former friends turn on her. *Saved!* brings up many issues of Christian culture and teen sexuality that are worth discussing. I had a feeling that watching a movie with Mandy Moore and Macaulay Culkin might stimulate more conversation than listening to Passport-2Purity lectures.

"What's the glue and paper for?" Katie asked as she walked over to the table in the corner of our room.

"It's for one of our activities. Pick two different-colored pieces of construction paper and glue them together. We need to let the glue dry and then we'll talk about it after dinner and the movie."

She pulled the supplies out of the bag and sat down at the table to pick her colors—light blue and yellow. Light blue has always been her favorite color. She glued the papers together and we headed to the hotel restaurant for dinner.

After we returned from dinner we stretched out on our bed and watched the movie.

Next up was the construction paper activity. I brought the

glued-together papers over to the bed and handed them to her.

"Katie, imagine one of these papers is you and the other is some guy you get into a relationship with. The glue is a special bond that's created when you decide to have sex. It's a bond that's designed to hold you together. But you're young and eventually one of you decides to break off the relationship. Now try to pull the papers apart."

She hadn't used a lot of glue, so the papers pulled apart relatively easily, but not without leaving pieces of each color on the other, along with a few rips and tears.

"Now pick out another piece of construction paper and glue it to the piece that represents you. We'll let it dry and then do this again in the morning." This time she picked red and glued it to her light blue paper.

The next morning we got up and went to breakfast in the Courtyard Restaurant. I ordered a side of bacon and a side of potatoes. She ordered pancakes. We made our plans for the day, figuring out which bus would take us to Powell's City of Books. But before we headed downtown, we had to finish the activity.

After we returned to our room, I handed her the red and blue glued-together papers. She knew what to do. She tried to pull them apart, but this time it was harder. The glue had set more overnight and there was just no way to separate them without seriously ripping them.

"So do you understand what happens when you have sex before you get married?" I asked.

"Yeah, it can get pretty messy." Katie picked at the red and yellow pieces of paper that were stuck to her light blue side.

"Yes, it can. But I hope you won't make as big of a mess as I did."

"Can we go to that bookstore now?"

#facingthetalk: Talk to your girl about bonding and how important it is to think about the long-term effects of significant relationships, including the risk of teen pregnancy. Be careful about communicating that her life will be ruined, that she'll be damaged goods or condemned to a terrible life if she chooses to have sex before marriage. It's just not true. Nobody is perfect.

Reflection. Perhaps I liked the construction paper activity because I still remembered every person I had chosen to have sex with when I was sexually active as a teen and young adult. Perhaps I liked it because it reminded me of the pain and sorrow I felt with every rejection, with every guy who would want to be close to me in the heat of the moment and the dark of night but distanced himself from me in the light of the day. There was no way of escaping my past. But I hoped this activity would help Katie choose a different path.

Life is messy. It just is. I don't know why we work so hard to be perfect and try to make it less messy. Sure, there are many messes we can avoid. But no matter what messes we get ourselves into, through our foolish choices or through the foolish choices of others, there's always hope for reconstruction. Why do we expect our girls to be picture perfect pieces of construction paper? Only God is perfect.

I didn't tell her about any of my messes. I was afraid that if I did, she might think it was okay to make messes and make even bigger messes than I had.

For some reason we've bought into the lie that if we're not perfect we will be condemned to a life of pain and sorrow. That's just not true. Jesus was perfect, yet he was fully acquainted with suffering and grief. Even Jesus had to die. But he was not condemned. He didn't stay dead. Like the hotel where Katie and I were staying, what some might want to condemn, others see as worth preserving and restoring.

Remember, God is with us to restore and redeem us. While we don't want our girls to make major mistakes, we have to let them make their own choices. Some of us learn best by learning things the hard way.

How-Not-To Sex Talk No. 3

It was the warmest mid-January weekend we'd had in a long time, with a low of fifty degrees and torrential rains that reached the Mt. Hood ski resort where we were staying thanks to a special package discount. We had planned to go snowboarding for Kelly's getaway. It wasn't in the budget, but Kelly, age fourteen, had saved her babysitting money so she could contribute. After she'd worked so hard to save, I could tell she was disappointed when the weather made snowboarding impossible. But there was nothing I could do about it. We made the best of it as we drove through the downpour up the Mt. Hood Highway.

We were listening to the Passport2Purity CDs as we drove. I'd given Kelly a notebook and pen and asked her to write down what she liked about the lessons and what she didn't like, along with any questions she might have. But there were times when I could barely see the road as the rain poured out of the clouds in buckets. We gave up trying to listen to the CDs so I could focus on driving and Kelly could help look for signs on the road. Finally, we arrived at The Resort at the Mountain and checked into our room.

I fumbled for the card key and pushed the door open with my shoulder. Our arms were overloaded with stuff from the car so we wouldn't have to make multiple trips in the downpour. I dropped my bag near the first bed, announcing, "I call this bed."

Kelly carefully placed her bags on the dresser near the foot of her bed and began to unpack and organize her space. I carried the bag of supplies for the activities over to the table near her bed and unpacked the pieces for the first activity of the day—a puzzle.

"Kelly, when you're done getting your stuff organized, I need you to try to put this puzzle together. You have ten minutes to work on the puzzle and see how much you can get done." The puzzle pieces were in a plastic baggie with no box or picture to guide her. The lid with the picture on it was hidden away to be used in the second part of the activity.

"While you work on the puzzle, I'll look into other fun things we can do since our snowboarding plans fell through. Do you have any ideas of what you might want to do?"

"We could just stay in the room and watch movies and read books," Kelly replied as she put her makeup bag, flat iron and toiletries in our shared bathroom.

"That sounds like a great idea. Since you're such a bookworm, I'm sure you packed a book or two. I'm not sure whether I did. I'll go check my bag." I left her to work on the puzzle while I searched for a book to read.

"Mom, where's the lid with the picture on it? I can't do it without the picture." Kelly rummaged through the bag of supplies.

"Well, you need to try. It's part of the activity. Just do your best. I'm sure you can figure some of it out." I sat down and put a few edge pieces together. She joined me reluctantly.

"Mom, this is really hard. I can't do it. I need to see the picture." Kelly liked to know how things were going to work out. Not having a plan seemed to cause her more anxiety than some kids.

"I understand it's hard. You only need to work on it for a few more minutes. You can do it." I set up the laptop so we could watch the movie *Saved!* before we went to bed.

She pushed the puzzle pieces around on the table for a few more minutes after getting most of the edges together. Kelly is good at puzzles, and she got almost all the pieces together. She has an amazing visual awareness and innate ability to see how small things fit together.

"Time's up." I walked over to the table. "You did great. Can you start to see what the picture is?"

"Well, I already figured out there are some sort of puppies or dogs in the grass—I can see the eyes and noses. And the green grass is obvious. Can I see the picture now so I can finish it?" Not only did she like to know how things were going to turn out, she didn't like to stop in the middle. I didn't realize how challenging this would be for her.

"We're going to take a break from the puzzle now. You can work on it again later. Let's watch a movie."

"Can we watch that movie *Saved!* that you brought?"

"Well, I was going to wait until after dinner to watch it. Let's watch something else and watch *Saved!* before bed."

After the movie was over, we had time to talk and work on the puzzle some more before dinner. I got the puzzle box lid from my bag and put it over on the table after scrambling the pieces to start over again.

"Let's see how long it takes us to put this together now that we have the picture," I said. Kelly grabbed the lid and set it up next to the space she'd cleared to work on the puzzle.

"Aw, these puppies are so cute," she said. She quickly put the edges together again and started working on the little puppy faces. I let her do the work herself but pointed out a few things.

The activity was intended to teach that you can't know God's plan for sex without having the Bible as your guide.

After she finished the puzzle, we headed out of our room for dinner.

We returned to our rooms and lounged on our beds for a while, chatting about love and relationships.

"Do you have any crushes right now?" I asked, propping my chin on my hands as I lay on my stomach facing her bed.

"Not really."

"Well, does anyone have a crush on you?" I knew of one crush I'd heard about from her younger sister but was waiting for her to tell me about it.

"No, but my friend Carly just came out as bi. She spent the night at our house last year. It kinda creeped me out."

"Why did it creep you out?"

"What if she was attracted to me? That would be weird."

I took a deep breath and shot up one of those arrow prayers again.

"Why would it be weird?" I asked.

"Because I don't like girls that way."

"How is it different from a boy you aren't interested in liking you?"

"I don't know. It just is."

"What would you do if she was attracted to you?"

"I don't know. Tell her I'm not attracted to girls? But what if people think I'm lesbian because of her?"

"You could go around wearing a T-shirt that says, 'I'm not a lesbian.' That would settle it for sure." I wasn't sure what to tell her, and sometimes when I'm anxious I make bad jokes.

"Mom! It's not funny. Doesn't the Bible say that God hates homosexuality?"

"Well, the Bible doesn't say a whole lot about homosexuality as a sexual orientation in the way we understand it today. Are you thinking about something from when we were reading through the Old Testament in family devotions last fall?"

"Yeah, I think there was a verse in the book of Leviticus about it being an abomination."

"You're right. That was a tough book to read, wasn't it?"

"Well, it was boring and I skipped a lot of it. Except the part about tattoos that Dad thought was so important. That was a fun discussion, but I don't think Karen convinced Dad of anything."

"You're right. Your dad still hates tattoos."

"But Karen did have a good point. We can't just read one verse and forget about the verses before and the verses after."

"Do you remember whether we talked about homosexuality when we read that part of Leviticus?"

"I don't remember."

"Me neither. But we can talk about it now. There are a lot of things in society around us that make us feel uncomfortable. I imagine that the early Israelites saw some pretty strange things as they encountered other societies. I think it's Leviticus 20 that talks about child sacrifice, adultery, men lying with men and incest."

"Yeah, and if God says it's wrong then it's wrong. Right?"

"Yes, that's one of the reasons we read through the whole Bible together as a family. God is still speaking to us today, and one of the ways he speaks is through the Bible. But we read the whole Bible because reading just one verse without understanding God's big story can lead us to some significant misunderstandings. And remember, we watch those Bibledex videos introducing the historical context so we can understand the big picture better.[5] Let's look at those Bible verses together."

I looked up Leviticus on my Bible app and we read chapter 20.

"So if the Bible says homosexuality is wrong, then what am I supposed to do about my friend?" Kelly asked. "Do I just stop being friends with her? And the Bible only talks about a man with a man as a bad thing, so what about lesbians?"

"Kelly, I don't have all the answers, but we can read more about it together when we get home. One thing I know is that some people interpret the various Bible passages about homosexual sex to mean that homosexual activity is a sin, not homosexual orientation. They say that being gay or lesbian is not a sin. So I don't think you have to stop being friends with her because of her being a lesbian. That wouldn't be very kind."

"I know, Mom. 'Be ye kind, one to another.' I memorized Ephesians 4:32 and you won't ever let me forget it. But there are some really mean people at school who call gays and lesbians names and even beat them up."

"Kelly, are you worried that someone might beat you up or call you names if they think you're a lesbian too?"

"Maybe, but nobody really notices me much at school because I'm shy. So I'm not too worried. I mostly hang out with the smart kids who are nice to me. But I heard in the news about some church that had signs that said, 'God hates fags,' and there was this kid who got beat up because of being gay. And last year a guy in Katie's class committed suicide because people were bullying him over his sexual orientation. I know what the Bible says, but I don't think God wants people to beat each other up or commit suicide."

"I don't think so either," I replied. "Fortunately, there aren't very many churches that go around with 'God hates fags' signs. Our pastor teaches that being gay or lesbian isn't a sin, and being attracted to someone of the same sex isn't a sin. But he teaches that God calls homosexuals to be celibate—to not have sex with same-sex partners."

"I think I heard someone say in youth group that God hates the sin but loves the sinner. I'm not sure how that works, but it feels like either way someone who's gay might feel hated. I can't imagine telling Carly, 'Oh, by the way, now that you're lesbian I hate what you do but I still love you as a friend.' That would just be totally weird."

"Yes, that would be weird. And Carly probably didn't just wake up one day and decide to be attracted to girls. Being attracted to someone isn't usually a conscious choice; it just kind of happens. But I don't think you have to worry about being a hater—Kelly, you're a very kind, smart, lovable young woman. In your life there might be both guys and gals who are attracted to you, and you won't return the feelings. Plus, there are lots of different types of people you could be attracted to. Just because you're attracted to someone doesn't mean you have to be in love with them. Long-term, loving relationships are way more complicated than mere attraction. You can't always choose who you're attracted to, but you can choose how you respond to that attraction."

"So gays and lesbians don't really have a choice about who they're attracted to?"

"I don't know. Everybody is different, but have you ever had a crush on somebody?"

"I don't really want to talk about that. Can we watch *Saved!* now?"

#facingthetalk: Do your best to be flexible and model grace in the midst of uncertainty. Be willing to talk about complexity without having all the answers. Join with your girl as she figures out what she thinks about the complexity around her.

Reflection. Things don't always turn out as planned. I planned to take Kelly on her How-Not-To getaway the summer after seventh grade, but neither of us was quite ready. Her two older sisters started their periods when they were in sixth and seventh grade. I thought for sure by the end of seventh grade Kelly would start. But she didn't. So I waited. I wanted our getaway to happen after she had officially started her journey into womanhood.

Kelly finally started her period after she turned fourteen, in the fall of ninth grade. I think her sisters and I were more anxious about when she would start than she was. It was no big deal to her, but Karen, Katie and I welcomed her to womanhood and celebrated with exuberant joy. It was all quite embarrassing to her. She asked us to calm down and even went to her room when I called to announce the news to my sister and mother. Kelly is an introvert and self-conscious about her body. She is also very smart and takes things seriously.

By the time I did my third How-Not-To getaway, I had started writing this book. Whenever I would tell people about my weekend getaways and how I intentionally talked to my girls about sex, they would often respond by saying, "Oh, you need to write a book about that. I would buy it." There was sometimes a hint of desperation in their voices. Writing a book gave me a different twist on this third getaway—I could ask Kelly to give me feedback! It was fun to get her input, and I think it motivated her to share more about things she found puzzling.

When we're faced with a puzzle, we often want to figure it out, get an answer, resolve the dilemma. Helping our children find their way in the world is a puzzle for sure, but it's an enigma, a mystery—not a jigsaw where their lives are rigidly predetermined by God and we just have to put the pieces together properly so that the picture is perfect in the end.

When my girls are faced with a puzzle, I'd rather they think about it critically rather than just go hunting for the answer, like searching for the jigsaw box top. Critical thinking is an important skill I hoped to help nurture in my girls. I wanted them to learn to analyze, evaluate, explain and reflect on their questions and the answers they found.

Before I went to seminary, I read through the whole Bible a few times and I had many questions. I hoped seminary would help answer at least some of them. In some ways it did, but in other ways it just led to more questions. I still find the Bible confusing when it comes to ideas about sex. Many men in the Old Testament have multiple wives, and then there's Hosea, who is instructed by God to marry a prostitute. In the New Testament Jesus forgives the adulterous woman and Paul encourages people to remain unmarried virgins forever. It's all complicated, and it's difficult to understand how it applies to our lives today.

Telling my girls they can experience lives of sexual integrity just by relying on the Bible as their guide—like a puzzle box top—doesn't seem fair. We need people to help us understand the Bible. We need community. We need family. We need love, not laws.

While my belief in a loving God revealed in Jesus Christ and experienced by the power of the Holy Spirit is very solid, beliefs like "God has a wonderful and detailed plan for your life; you can know it and have complete confidence that everything will turn out right in the end if you read your Bible and obey everything in it" and "God said it; I believe it; that settles it" are losing power in my life.

But this idea that God has a picture-perfect plan for life is very appealing.

How-Not-To Sex Talk No. 4

Kimberly, age thirteen, had carried the gift bag from the car to the hotel. It was a hot day in Redding, but that was to be expected.

"Mom, can I wear my ring?"

"Well, you wouldn't want to lose it on a waterslide, so let's wait until later to open it."

We unpacked the car, put on our bathing suits and headed out for the afternoon. We arrived at the waterslide park for our outing and tried to avoid frying in the sun. One of the benefits of living in Seattle with fair-skinned children was not having to put sunscreen on every day. Rainy days do have their benefits. But in California, we had to be careful. We spent the first few minutes at the waterslide park protecting our skin with SPF 70. After we were fully coated, we climbed up to the giant serpentine slides and waited in the hot sun.

Kimberly was used to waiting. She had been thinking about this getaway and her special ring for seven years.

"When can I have my ring?" she asked while we were waiting to go down the corkscrew slide.

"Later tonight in the hotel room. I promise you can open it then."

We waited in the long lines a few more times and then left the water park. We went to dinner and an evening church service, then headed back to the hotel to watch *Saved!* Her sisters had already given her a sneak preview of what to expect this weekend. Both Katie and Kelly had told her about watching this movie.

"Can I have my ring now?" The door had barely closed behind us as we returned to our hotel room.

"Do you want to open it before or after the movie?"
"Before."

I handed her the gift bag and watched her open it.

"Kimberly, this ring is a gift from your dad and me because we love you very much. If you want it to represent your commitment to wait until marriage to have sex, we support that, but it's your choice. What this ring represents for us is our commitment to love you no matter what."

"I know, Mom. I know you love me."

"Your dad and I think waiting until marriage to express your love for another through sexual intercourse is a good idea, but ultimately it's your choice. We will love you no matter who you love, no matter how you love and no matter when you love. We will always love you no matter what."

Kimberly put the ring on her finger and gave me a hug.

"Thanks, Mom. I love my ring. It's beautiful."

"Yes, it is. You chose well. And you're beautiful too. I bet you have lots of boys in school interested in you."

"I don't know. I don't really pay much attention to boys. Most of them are stupid." She twisted her new ring around her finger a few times.

"I'm sure that's not true. Well, okay—junior high boys can be kind of awkward. I remember when I was in junior high . . ."

"Mom! Not another story about when you were a teenager! Can we start the movie now?"

"Okay, let's get our pajamas on and then we'll watch it."

> **#facingthetalk:** Encourage your girl to wait until marriage to have sex but commit to loving her no matter what. Remind her that ultimately it's her choice about love and sex. Show her how loved she is. Explain how sex is a powerful expression of committed love.

Reflection. When I got the first ring for Karen, it wasn't strictly a purity ring. We gave it to her around the time of the getaway, but we gave it as a birthday gift to express our love for her. We told her that if she wanted to use the ring as a symbol to represent her desire to remain a virgin until marriage, we would support that. At age twenty-one Karen remains an unmarried virgin, but she lost her ring years ago. I thought we might find it when we cleaned out her room after she moved to college, but she must have lost it at school or a sporting event. We bought Karen a new ring and she continues to wear it as a reminder of our commitment to love her and as a symbol of her desire to wait until marriage to have sex.

We decided to let Katie, Kelly and Kimberly pick their own rings. Kimberly started shopping for hers soon after she started her period. She had been anticipating her turn to get a special ring ever since we gave Karen hers. She wanted a ring with her birthstone. One day when we were out shopping, she found the perfect ring. I let her try it on and it was perfect.

I bought the ring for her that day but made her wait until our getaway to give it to her. She was used to waiting.

Kimberly is fifteen as I write this. She has decided to wear the ring as a symbol of her desire to wait until marriage to have sex, but she also sees it as a reminder of our love for her.

When our girls were young and would threaten to run away, we told them it was their choice and that we would love them no matter where they lived. I wondered if we could do the same thing with their sexuality. Could we tell them we would love them no matter who they chose to love? No matter how they chose to love? No matter when they chose to have sex? Yes, we decided. We could and we would.

By the time it was Kimberly's turn to have the How-Not-To talk, I'd been through enough drama with my older girls to know I'd never have a picture-perfect family. With Kimberly being the youngest of four whose mother was writing a book on talking to girls about sex, you can imagine how many conversations she had to endure. Even though talking about sex is commonplace in our home, she was still looking forward to her special getaway. It was tradition. It was important.

But it wasn't virginity that made these getaways important. The purpose was not to safeguard my daughters like perfect roses to be presented to their future spouses. My purpose was always to facilitate bonding, communicate their worth and help them make wise choices about their sexuality. Sometimes that purpose was clouded with fear on my part. But even in the midst of my own storms, I wanted my daughters to know they were loved and to know how to express their sexuality in a way that communicated how valuable and lovable they were. I didn't want them to go looking for love in all the wrong places like I had.

While communicating my unconditional love was important, I also knew my love was not enough. Their dad's love was not enough. Even God's love was not enough—God's love isn't much help when you stop believing in God, and most young people go through times of doubting and unbelief during adolescence. I wanted my daughters to learn to love themselves. Not some ideal spiritual self, illusory perfect-ten physical self or supersmart, high-achieving self. I wanted them to love their real, actual selves, imperfections and all.

One of the keys to a healthy sexual ethic is loving others as we love ourselves. While in Christian circles we often focus on the "loving others" part of the equation, we sometimes forget that loving ourselves is a key to loving others. I'm not talking about narcissism here. Narcissism is characterized by extreme selfishness and excessive interest in one's physical appearance. I'm talking about a healthy love of self that's rooted in an accurate estimate of oneself and an acceptance of limitations, differences and weaknesses along with talents, abilities and strengths as part of what it means to be human.

Jesus showed us what it is to be fully human. Being like Jesus does not mean conforming to an elusive ideal of purity or beauty, but rather conforming to the image of God. And the only way to be conformed to God's image is to be shaped and formed by God. That's what it means to be human—to be shaped and formed by forces outside of ourselves. We were designed to be shaped and formed by God, and Jesus made a way for that to happen through the indwelling of the Holy Spirit. We are also shaped and formed by our attachments—to God and other people. If the people we bond with are bonded with God, then God will be a stronger influence in our lives. Family and Christian community are the glue that help us bond well with Jesus.

While I knew my girls might have seasons of doubt and unbelief, I also knew that encouraging a strong attachment to God was one of my most important tasks. It was a more important task than protecting their virginity.

Too often we treat purity pledges and purity rings as if they have some magical power—as if our girls can say the pledge or put on the ring and be protected as if by a charm or spell from the evils of this oversexualized world. Or we look to our faith to protect them. If we just get them to attend youth group and read their Bible and say the right prayers, they will be safe. If they can have a supernatural encounter with God, then everything will be fine. But even Jesus doesn't promise such protection: "I have told you these things, so that in me you may have peace. In this world you will have trouble. But take heart! I have overcome the world" (John 16:33).

We all face disappointment. It's part of life. Even life with God. Disappointment often leads to discouragement, and discouragement to despair. Our girls will face disappointment in their lives. And they might even disappoint us a few times along the way. Will we fear disappointment and try to avoid it, or will we face disappointment with courage and grace? The opposite of discouragement is encouragement and the opposite of despair is faith.

Let's encourage our girls with faith and hope—faith that they will make wise choices, and hope that they will find God's peace in the midst of life's struggles.

Purity vs. Virginity

What do we hope for our girls? What is our desire for our conversations with them about sex? One of my desires was to help my girls make different choices than I had made, but that is a very reactionary motivation. You have a different story. Maybe you waited until marriage to have sex and want the same for your girls. Maybe you had an abortion and hope your girls are never faced with that decision. Regardless of the starting point, there are many good reasons to talk to our girls about sex.

Remember, one of the primary tasks of adolescence is identity development. From age thirteen to about nineteen, adolescents work to resolve conflicts and confusion that develop as their primary identity moves from that of a member of a family to a member of society. They continue to develop their understanding of manhood and womanhood and experiment with gender roles. A full 90 percent of teens report sexual debut by age twenty. That statistic is only slightly lower in Christian communities, where 80 to 85 percent of young people report sexual debut by age twenty. Six to 8 percent of girls report experiences with someone of the same sex during adolescence, though most still choose hetero-sexual orientation at this stage.

Adolescence is sometimes defined as a time of moving from a state of dependence to a state of independence. We often mark this time as corresponding with the teen years, typically cutting it off at age eighteen or graduation from high school. Some argue that adolescence now extends to age twenty-five since young people are still somewhat dependent in their early twenties, especially with increasing college costs and other eco-nomic changes society is experiencing.

I define adolescence as that period of individuation when young people are discovering their unique identity and figuring out where they fit in the family and other social systems. This is an intense time because young people are experiencing signif-icant physiological changes as well as important sociological changes. They may experience decreased desire to spend time with family members and increased desire to relate to a romantic partner. They are learning to manage physical and emotional intimacy in relationships, mostly through modeling.

These factors raise a number of questions for us to consider as parents. What kind of role models are we offering our girls? How are we managing physical and emotional intimacy in our family relationships? What are their friends modeling for them? How much exposure to media messages are they getting? What's a healthy balance?

The connection between developing a stable sense of self and establishing a healthy sexuality is significant. We exist as sexual beings—we cannot separate our sense of self from our embodied experience. In addition to our physically assigned sex, we have issues of gender identity. Remember that sex refers to biological differences—sex organs and other physical factors—while gender refers to the characteristics a society connects with masculinity or femininity. A person's sex as male or female is a biological fact that varies little across time and cultures, but what that sex means in terms of gender roles as a man or a woman in society differs across cultures and across time. In a world where gender roles are constantly and quickly changing, it's normal for girls to wrestle with role confusion and to experiment with gender roles in ways that are foreign to us.

Imposing cultural stereotypes, even Christian cultural stereotypes, of what it means to be feminine onto our girls may not be helpful. They are constantly being bombarded by the media (even by the church) with the idea that a "bombshell" or a "hot chick" is the ideal feminine gender role, and they are incessantly pressured to fit into someone else's mold. One of our primary jobs as parents (and parental figures) is to help our girls think critically about the gender role messages they receive from society and teach them how to be renewed in their thinking. Our hope is that they will choose to conform to the image of Christ, not the image of a Victoria's Secret model.

The big questions our girls are asking themselves and wrestling with in the context of their social relationships are "Who am I?" and "Who can I be?" Their motivation is toward integrity and fidelity in their identity—there is something deep within that drives them to be known for who they truly are—yet they are in the process of discovering this for themselves.

During this stage of development we can help our girls discover their true selves and wrestle with questions of gender role and identity development in the context of a safe, loving and accepting community. Dominating the discussion with issues of virginity limits the conversation and creates an in-out proposition that can potentially be harmful to our daughters' authentic selves. Once they cross the line out of the virginity circle, they may feel like they have lost themselves in the process and wander off into a world defined by sexual objectification, losing far more than their virginity.

In order to help our girls with these questions of identity, we need to help them understand the connection between purity and integrity. Perhaps unintentionally, through a focus on purity pledges, we have too narrowly defined purity as virginity. While we may not explicitly communicate this, our girls often hear the message that if they do not remain a virgin until marriage, all is lost. This creates a sense of being in or out, a culture of us versus them—it's very black and white. Yes, sex within the confines of a loving marriage relationship is a healthy goal to present to our young people. But I wonder if equating purity with virginity is just as much a sexualization of our girls as the popular media messages. Some curriculums do discuss purity in broader terms, but by asking our girls to sign a pledge to remain a virgin until marriage, we often obscure the rest of the message in the process.

So what does it truly mean to be pure? Ideas of purity, holiness, cleanliness and sanctification are prevalent in the Old and New Testaments. By the time Jesus came on the scene, Jewish religious leaders had established some pretty strict rules regarding purity—which Jesus countered by saying that purity was a matter of the heart (Matthew 15:19).

The word "pure" is defined in the dictionary as:

- not mixed or adulterated with any other substance or material: cars can run on pure alcohol; the jacket was pure wool.

- without any extraneous and unnecessary elements: the romantic notion of pure art devoid of social responsibility.

- free of any contamination: the pure, clear waters of Montana.

- wholesome and untainted by immorality, especially that of a sexual nature: our fondness for each other is pure and innocent.

When I first started these purity talks with my girls, I didn't know exactly why purity was so important except that it was what all good Christian moms expected of their daughters, and it was how all good Christian girls were expected to be—pure and innocent until their wedding day. I had memorized 1 Thessalonians 4:1-8 when I was single and committed to abstaining from sex until marriage, even though I wasn't a virgin. I didn't have *The Message* version of the Bible back then, but I like the way it presents this passage:

> One final word, friends. We ask you—*urge* is more like it—that you keep on doing what we told you to do to please God, not in a dogged religious plod, but in a living, spirited dance. You know the guidelines we laid out for you from the Master Jesus. God wants you to live a pure life.
>
> Keep yourselves from sexual promiscuity.
>
> Learn to appreciate and give dignity to your body, not abusing it, as is so common among those who know nothing of God.
>
> Don't run roughshod over the concerns of your brothers and sisters. Their concerns are God's concerns, and *he* will take care of them. We've warned you about this before. God hasn't invited us into a disorderly, unkempt life but into something holy and beautiful—as beautiful on the inside as the outside.
>
> If you disregard this advice, you're not offending your neighbors; you're rejecting God, who is making you a gift of his Holy Spirit. (1 Thessalonians 4:1-8, *The Message*)

This passage was written to Christians in a society where sexual immorality was often practiced in the context of the mystery religions. People had sexual relations in order to increase fertility, as an act of worship of false gods whom they believed were responsible for blessing their crops, their flocks and their own ability to bear offspring. The context of 1 Thessalonians has more to do with who we're worshiping than whether to kiss on the first date. It's about our identity as embodied spiritual beings who are created to worship the one true God. We are created to be dedicated to God—God is king. When we serve other things with our sexuality we are rejecting God's authority. Our truest selves long to worship, and if our passions are not rightly directed, we will worship things other than God. Helping our girls discover their true selves in relationship to God is important, and helping them see how their choices regarding sex relate to worshiping God is helpful—but what if they reject God?

Young people often wrestle with faith in God and reject God's authority during this critical developmental stage in life. David Kinnaman reports in *You Lost Me: Why Young Christians are Leaving the Church* that 59 percent of young people with a Christian background drop out of church for some time.[6] While it's true that our sexuality is tied to worship, requiring young people to make a pledge to God may not be the best way to help them discover their true identity as beings created to worship God. When they doubt their faith or reject God for a time, the purity pledge goes out the window. Instead, our task is to guide them in the process of discovering their authentic selves—that they're someone who is created in the image of God.

Many of us like the idea that inside us there's a God-shaped hole that only God can fill. I prefer the idea from the lullaby I sang for my girls when they were young, that we are handmade by God, each of us unique in all our ways, designed to praise God all of our days.

Our authentic self, our true identity, is found in worshiping God. As we help our girls discover their true identity and develop a healthy sense of self, we hope they will recognize the reality that they are created to worship God and will choose to express that worship through their sexuality. The image of God is stamped on them at birth—or perhaps conception—and we can help them discover it. This image is not removed from them if they cross the line of virginity before marriage. It may be obscured by messages of shame, but God's image remains firmly fixed in their heart of hearts. Until they recognize this truth, we must handle them with care—after all, they are handmade by God; they are God's special creations entrusted to our care.

Even if our girls reject God and reject us for a time, helping them ask the questions "Who am I?" and "Who can I be?" will guide them to discover their true selves. I don't always know how to do this well, but I try to ask my daughters questions that get them thinking about who they are and who they want to be. I wish someone had helped me ask those questions when I was an adolescent. I allowed others to define who I was. I have struggled with discovering my authentic self ever since. There are many forces out there seeking to define our girls, to lure them away from finding their identity in Christ and participating in God's kingdom. How will we help them discern who they are? How will we help them choose who defines them?

7

Talking Topics

Ages Thirteen to Seventeen

We hadn't seen each other for years. Anna and I were best of friends once. She was in my wedding and I was in hers. She was there when my first daughter was born, helping me through labor and delivery with her skills as a massage therapist. She was the kind of friend who always gave good health advice, knew all about manners and looked put-together even when she was going out to exercise. We'd lost touch over the years but reconnected one summer when our family was vacationing in Santa Cruz. We arrived in town and she offered to take my girls to the beach while my husband and I settled into my stepbrother's apartment. He was out of town and let us stay in his place while he was gone.

Anna's kids were younger than mine—my girls were fifteen, thirteen, eleven and nine at the time—but they all had fun to-gether anyway. After Anna brought the girls back from the beach, she pulled me aside to speak privately.

Makeup

"May I teach your girls how to put on makeup?" Anna asked with a smile.

I almost shouted, "*Yes, please!*" in response to her offer. "Sure," I said. "You know I'm not into makeup. What are you thinking?"

"Well, I noticed they're using a lot of black eyeliner around their eyes."

"I know! Ken really doesn't like that look. He says it looks like they have a black eye. It's not my favorite either, but I don't have much to offer them as an alternative. I prefer the next-to-nothing end of the spectrum, but there has to be a happy medium. Your makeup always looks good, so thanks for offering to help. What do you need from me?"

"Nothing. I'll stop by the drugstore and pick up a few things and then I can show them some options when you come to my house for dinner."

"That sounds lovely. I'll let them know."

We headed back to the apartment and cleaned the sand out of our toes.

"Girls, Anna wants to show you some tricks on doing your makeup." I hoped they would be interested.

"I know how to do my makeup already," Katie replied as she sat down on her cousin's superhero bed.

"Well, Katie, you know how your dad feels about all that black eyeliner you wear. It might be nice to learn some other options. Anna always looks nice and she's going to buy some makeup for you to try on."

"Oooh, makeup! Will she get some fun colors?" Kelly chimed in enthusiastically. It didn't surprise me that Kelly was interested. She had just started wearing makeup and it was still new and exciting for her.

"I'm sure it will be fun. It's very nice of her to offer to do this for you, so please be respectful, even if she doesn't get the colors you like."

"Do I get to do makeup too?" Kimberly asked.

"That's up to you. If you want to watch or put some on that's fine, but it's just for fun. You don't get to wear makeup every day until you're older."

Kimberly had just finished fourth grade. We only let our girls wear a little blush or lip gloss at that age, and just on special occasions. We let them wear eye makeup around sixth or seventh grade. Karen and Katie had been wearing makeup for a while by then and I wasn't very excited about how they did it. Neither Ken nor I liked their look, but we didn't know what to do about it. I hoped a makeup session with Anna would help steer them in a different direction without inciting an argument over how much was too much eyeliner.

A few hours later we arrived at her house. Anna had been a busy shopper—she'd purchased makeup and some teen magazines. I wasn't a fan of magazines like *Seventeen* or *Teen Vogue*, but I trusted Anna's judgment. She had the makeup and magazines set out on the table near the kitchen.

"Hi, girls! Go ahead and have a seat at the table and take a look at the magazines. Pick out your favorite makeup look from the pictures—not your favorite pop star, your favorite makeup look. Look at the eyes and cheeks and lips. When I'm done cutting up the vegetables, we'll talk about it and then practice putting on some makeup." Anna was always the cheery one.

Karen and Katie started looking through the magazines and talking about *Gossip Girl* since Blake Lively was on the cover, while Kelly started picking out makeup to try. I liked Blake

Lively's look, even though I didn't like *Gossip Girl*. Some people get upset about violence and language on TV shows, but the ones that bother me the most are shows that portray women as catty, petty and gossipy.

"Okay, girls, Anna asked you to pay attention to makeup, not talk about TV shows."

"Yeah, and we're not allowed to watch *Gossip Girl* anyway!" Kelly waited her turn to look at the magazines.

Kimberly wasn't interested in the magazines or the makeup. While her older sisters were complaining about how they weren't allowed to watch *Gossip Girl* and defending Blake Lively because of her role in *The Sisterhood of the Traveling Pants* movies, Kimberly tugged on my sleeve to get my attention.

"Mom, can I go in the pool?" Kimberly asked.

"Only if your dad will watch you." I looked over at Ken to see if he was up for it.

Ken nodded and took the younger kids out back to play.

Anna finished chopping the vegetables and then joined the girls at the table. I stayed out of the way but close enough to learn a little something for myself.

Anna let each girl show the image she had chosen and then explained how that particular look was achieved. She was brilliant when it came to understanding how adding a little shading here, a little white liner there and a little blending all over worked to accomplish a certain look. She explained how some techniques made your eyes look bigger and how heavy black eyeliner made your eyes look smaller. She talked to them about different face shapes, eye placement and lip sizes. It was all a foreign language to me. But I was grateful that Anna was helping my girls to see themselves as they really were—not as they imagined they would be based on some picture in a magazine.

Anna took each girl to a mirror and showed her how to do things with makeup she'd never known before. Whenever I talked to my girls about makeup, it always turned dramatic. She taught them art rather than drama. They each emerged from the bathroom with a fresh new look that suited their coloring and their features.

It was magic.

I watched but I didn't really learn much—it's more than sensitive skin that keeps me from putting on makeup. You know how some people have a knack for decorating or a green thumb or can play music by ear—and others don't? Well, I'm one of the others when it comes to makeup. It's still a mystery to me even after all the makeup demonstrations I've endured to help my friends start their home businesses. Some women just aren't born that way.

But many are. We could blame the media and *America's Next Top Model* for the fascination our girls have with makeup and dressing up, but that wouldn't be entirely fair. It's true—movies, TV, magazines and other media images influence our view of what is beautiful, and being concerned about how we look is somewhat culturally conditioned. But many women are inherently and naturally interested in these things.

Reflection. Looking back, I realize that some of my discomfort with makeup and fashion was a result of a lack of interest. I wasn't interested in those things even when I was a teen. I was also influenced by some of my mentors when I was a young Christian who taught that dressing up and wearing makeup was worldly. Godly women didn't care about such things. That was easy for me to accept because I didn't care much about them anyway.

I didn't train Katie or Kelly to be interested in fashion or makeup—but they both are. I didn't train Karen to be interested in sports—but she enjoys playing softball and running around with her friends more than she cares about fashion or makeup. I'm still trying to figure Kimberly out—some days it seems like she's working hard to be different from all of her sisters in one way or another. It's a strange thing to have four very different girls. I wonder if parents of multiple children of the same gender are less likely to hold gender-based stereotypes.

When I look at my girls, I see them all as beautiful. (I am biased, of course.) But they are all very different in their tastes for clothing, hairstyles, makeup and how much time they take to get ready to go somewhere. They're different in whether they prefer sports or reading, spending time with friends or being alone, and an infinite number of other ways. Plus they all have their own beauty standard that matches their interests and per-sonality. One might be more influenced by her internal sense of being put together, another by what she likes on people in the media, and another by what her small group leader at church wears. All of these inform their sense of what is beautiful and what is acceptable to wear.

> **#facingthetalk:** Help girls know their unique style. Beauty is only one of many praiseworthy attributes. Help them feel safe in their own skin. Be sure to notice other attributes such as strength, intelligence, com-mon sense and so on. Help your girl recognize why she likes certain things. Help her ask good questions about herself and the beauty stan-dards of the media, her friends and the church.

Dating Rules

Even though Derek had moved away, he and his family occa-sionally returned to our neighborhood for summer barbecues and Christmas and New Years parties. He was a senior and Karen was a sophomore, but they had lived next door to each other since she was two. They reconnected during a neighborhood barbecue, then left with their friends to walk the street and hang out away from the little kids and adults. Teenagers are like that. It's part of their process of differentiation—one of the ways they keep saying, "I am not a kid, and I am not you!"

The usual topics of discussion arose about what their friends were up to and what classes they were taking and who they were going to homecoming with this year. Karen jokingly lamented that she didn't have a date or any close friends that she was really looking forward to going with.

She saw Derek's kindness bubble up into his bright blue eyes as he blurted out, "If you don't get a date, I'll go with you."

"Cool," she responded nonchalantly. "That would be fun."

Her first thought when she'd seen him on this visit was, *When did he get cute?* She tried not to betray her interest in going to homecoming with him, wishing he'd just asked her outright. This was all rather awkward anyway since he went to a different school now.

The first thought that crossed my mind when she told me of his kindness was, *But he's not a Christian. And I think he might smoke pot.* I feel like such a hypocrite at times. When I was seventeen, I wasn't a Christian and I smoked pot! But while my choices at that age definitely affected my future, they did not determine my future in a predictable way. Would I discourage my daughter from going to homecoming with a nice boy out of fear? Would I judge and label this kind young man whose father committed suicide when he was a toddler, who was courageously raised by a single mother alone for most of his young life? Would I pronounce a terrible fate on him, calling him no good—at least not good enough for my daughter—because he might be engaging in risky behavior?

My generous thoughts overshadowed my fears and I responded, "I bet that would be fun! That was kind of him to offer to go with you. What are you going to do?"

I was also tempted to ask, "Do you think he's interested in you romantically?" But I resisted. I tried not to ask that question too often or too early with my girls' cross-gender friendships. These friendships are oversexualized enough in the media and among their peers. They didn't need that pressure at home too.

"I'm sure it would be fun, but I'd rather have a date," she said matter-of-factly as she began to twirl the red curls hanging over her collarbone.

"Dinner's almost ready," Ken called from the kitchen.

"Well, why don't you ask him to be your date?" I suggested as I began to clear my seminary books and papers off the table for dinner.

"No, Mom! That wouldn't be a real date." She was emphatic, putting her hands on her hips and standing firm in her convictions.

I stopped clearing the table and looked at her intently. I didn't want this to turn into an argument, but I felt it was a great opportunity to help her think about what she believed about dating and friendship between women and men.

"Well, he offered to go with you and I imagine you two would have fun together. I'm sure you'll make a good decision." I put my hand on her shoulder as she returned to twirling her long red curls. She didn't squirm away from my touch this time, but just stood there thinking. I left her to her thoughts and returned to the kitchen to help Ken serve dinner.

A few nights later, we both had a stack of books on the cherry wood table. Karen was doing her homework and I was working on my online seminary class work. At least we were starting off the school year right keeping up with our assignments. Karen's freckled face was shadowed by a grimace as she opened her math book. Math never was her favorite subject.

"Mom, can I switch math classes?" she asked, tapping her pencil on the notebook paper.

I raised my finger to indicate I needed a minute. I quickly finished the paragraph I was writing.

I looked up from my computer and asked, "Why? What's wrong?"

"Mr. Pinter is really mean and he's not a very good teacher. I don't understand anything we're doing so far." Her normally soft blue eyes sparked as she flipped through the pages of her math text.

"But you've only had him for a week! He can't be that bad." I crossed my arms, anticipating a fight.

I wasn't going to let her off the hook that easily. Our philosophy of education involved taking responsibility for teaching our children and viewing the public school teachers as those we had selected to teach them. We instructed our girls to respect the education system and to work within its bounds. I didn't mind hearing Karen's complaints or helping her process her feelings and make a wise decision about what to do, but I wasn't going to make that decision for her or go to the school and demand anything on her behalf.

"But, Mom, all my friends say he's a terrible teacher. He's the football coach and only likes the boys in the class. He doesn't even think girls can be good at math!" She was sitting up straight now, ready to fight.

I clenched my jaw. The mother bear in me wanted to run up

to the school right then and there and demand the teacher be fired immediately. But it was evening and the school was closed.

"Has he done anything in your class that made you feel that way or is it just rumors you've heard? And have you talked to your counselor about this?" I replied as calmly as I could.

"It's just what I've heard, but I can already tell he doesn't like me." Sadness washed out the fire in her eyes as she picked up her pencil and started working on her math problems. "I haven't talked to my counselor yet, 'cause she'll just tell me I have to stick it out."

I let the subject drop and picked up my post-Christendom book to continue my studies.

Karen fidgeted her way through a page of math problems before pushing back the chair to go get a snack. I looked up from my reading as she returned to the table, shuffling her books around to start working on a new subject.

At that moment I decided to change subjects too. "Has anyone asked you to homecoming?" I wanted to bite my tongue as soon as the words left my mouth.

"No, Mom. And I wish you would stop asking." The fire flamed in her eyes again.

"Why don't you just ask somebody?" I shifted in my chair as I tried to recover from my mistake.

"Mom, I don't want to ask somebody. I want to be asked." She pulled her history book toward her on the table and leaned it up between us to create a safe boundary.

"There's nothing wrong with girls asking guys. It's just a dance, and who says you can't be the one doing the asking?" My mini-lecture fell on deaf ears as Karen dove into her history book, ignoring my every word.

My anxiety got the best of me a little over a week later when

I asked that dreaded question again.

"Did anyone ask you to homecoming?"

The hopeful lilt in my voice barely covered my anxiety as I twisted the hair that fell over my shoulder. I think Karen picked up the habit from me.

She was sitting on the tan leather couch, reading *Beowulf* for English class.

"I decided to go with Derek." The glint in her eye betrayed the straight-faced expression she adopted so I wouldn't get too excited for her. To me it felt as if she was the one who'd just slain a monster instead of Beowulf!

"I'm so excited for you!" I nearly jumped with glee, but I kept my feet planted on the hardwood floor so I wouldn't scare her off from the rest of the conversation. "When did you decide that?"

"Oh, we were texting the other day and I decided to take him up on his offer. Can you help me download and print the permission form since he goes to a different school?"

"Of course. I'd be glad to help."

#facingthetalk: Be careful about reinforcing romantic ideals that cast women as powerless recipients of whatever men have to offer.

Look for opportunities to talk about dating, romance and gender ideals—what do you believe about the role of women in dating and marriage and how do you want to communicate those ideas?

Reflection. When I was younger, traditions made me feel safe. They made things more predictable. Children of alcoholics and abuse victims often find solace in orderliness and routine. Because Karen was the eldest, my mean-mad-mom days likely affected her more than her sisters. Traditions made her feel safe too.

But some traditions just don't make sense to me. Why does a society built on democracy still celebrate the crowning of kings and queens at homecoming dances? What is so alluring about the king and queen, prince and princess ideal anyway? The princess line of Bibles, movies such as *The Princess Diaries* and the parade of Disney princesses through the years all play on this theme. Do all young girls want to be princesses? What does it mean to be treated like a princess? What does it mean to *be* a princess? While princesses are born into royalty, most of the stories include a romantic element that communicates that the primary role of the princess is to marry the right prince—to be chosen. Movies like Disney's *Brave* are challenging older fairy-tale notions, but don't we all want to be desired?

A part of me hoped someone would ask Karen to go to home-coming. I wanted her to feel the joy of being desired, of being sought after, of being accepted in this crazy, messed-up world we live in. But I also wanted to empower her to be the desiring one, the seeking one, the accepting one. We all need to feel loved and accepted in the world—boys as well as girls.

How do we help our daughters develop a healthy sense of worth? How do we help them feel beloved? This is something I struggle with often. My prayer is that the love they experience at home and in their church community will help them know how deeply they are loved and accepted by God and by those who know them best.

Sex on TV

"Dad won't let us watch *Glee* next week!"

"Mom, did you get my text?"

"Mom, text me or call me!"

Kelly, age fifteen, texted me in a panic after watching the

latest episode of *Glee* with her sisters and her dad. *Glee* is a network TV teen drama series featuring characters involved in a high school glee club.

I didn't see her texts until after I arrived in Portland. I was only there for a couple of days, but I sensed the urgency. I knew how much she loved watching *Glee*.

"Oh no! Why won't he let you watch it?" I replied late that night.

"Because it's all about sex."

"Oh. Okay. But why are you texting me about this? You need to respect your dad."

"It's not fair. It's my favorite show."

"I'm sure your dad has good reasons. We can talk about this when I get home."

When I returned from Portland, Kelly bombarded me almost immediately. When was I going to talk to her dad about *Glee*? Why couldn't she watch it? She didn't want to skip an episode because it would mess up the whole story line. She was just going to watch it on the computer by herself anyway, so what did it matter what Dad said?

Kelly cares a lot about following the rules, so when she breaks them, she usually lets us know. She desperately wanted her dad to change his mind so she could watch the next episode of *Glee* without breaking any rules. Even if it meant breaking the rule of trying to pit one parent against the other.

Ken and I have tried to follow that timeworn parenting advice about presenting a unified front—talking about our differences in private, coming to some level of agreement and then presenting that position to the kids. But the reality is that most of the time we aren't very good at it. And I'm not convinced that husbands and wives dealing with disagreements in private is all that helpful for our children. In some ways it creates a false world where being married is all peace, joy and harmony. It sets up an ideal where the two-become-one theology means two people have to become more alike than different in order to be well-adjusted and raise well-adjusted kids.

However, this was one instance where processing privately seemed like the best course of action.

After I threw my duffle bag into my messy closet to be unpacked the next day, I asked Ken to come talk with me privately. We live in a house with an open floor plan, so "privately" usually means behind closed doors in our bedroom.

"What did I do wrong now?" Ken asked as he closed the bedroom door behind him.

"Nothing. I just need to talk with you about *Glee* and I don't want to talk in front of Kelly. She's too emotionally wrapped up in this to listen right now. I haven't seen the preview for the next episode, so will you explain why they're banned from watching next week?" I straightened the sheets and comforter before I sat on the edge of the bed. It hadn't been made since before I left for Portland.

"Well, there's so much sexual content in that show that I don't think they should be watching it at all. They convinced me to let them watch it because they really like the music and it is somewhat entertaining. But next week's episode is all about high schoolers having sex for the first time. We don't want our girls having sex while they're dating and in high school, and *Glee* glorifies and romanticizes such experiences. It's not good." Ken sat down on the edge of the bed with me after I finished straightening things up.

"We let them watch TV shows and movies with violence in them even though we don't want them to go out and kill people.

How is this different?" I totally ignored all that advice I learned in couples' counseling about listening to the other person's point of view, showing empathy and working together to come up with a solution. Instead, I pulled out the big guns and tried to start a fight.

"That's different. In the movies and shows we watch with violence there are clearly good guys and bad guys. And the good guys win. *Glee* is blurring the line between right and wrong. By showing teen sex in a positive light—even gay teen sex—they're promoting an agenda that's not God's agenda. Teen sex is risky. And gay sex is just wrong. I don't think we need to expose our girls to thinking that teen sex, gay or straight, is something to be celebrated or embraced."

"You're right. Teen sex is risky. But I'm not convinced that keeping them from watching an episode of *Glee* is going to prevent them from being exposed to such ideas. They're already exposed to those ideas in school and in the music they listen to. It's part of teen culture and *Glee* is merely illustrating what exists in society around us. I show our girls a movie that deals with teen sex when I take them on our weekend getaways. Watching shows like this with them gives us an opportunity to talk about these things."

Ken wasn't convinced. "You know I'm not comfortable talking about this stuff with them. And it's really not that complicated. Sex before marriage is wrong, and gay sex is wrong. What more do we need to say?"

"Not everyone thinks as logically as you do. Your software engineer's brain sees most things in binary terms—it's either black or white, right or wrong. If just telling teens that sex before marriage is wrong worked, we wouldn't have church kids having sex as often as everybody else. It's complicated. That's why I talk to the girls about it so much." My heart was starting to beat louder in my chest. There are some topics I always get fired up about.

"I still don't think we should let them watch *Glee* next week." Ken started to get up from the edge of the bed and head for the door.

"Wait," I said. I remembered some of our couples' counseling advice and tried to think of a compromise. "How about if we watch it first and then decide together whether they're allowed to watch it? It might not be as bad as you think." I reached for his hand before he grabbed the doorknob.

"Okay. We can watch it together later this week." He gave my hand a loving squeeze before we headed back downstairs.

Reflection. While I understood Ken's reasons for reacting to the *Glee* episode preview the way he did, I wasn't comfortable with his ban. In my experience, one way to ensure conflict is to take an extreme position on a controversial topic without first understanding where the other person stands. This tends to promote a culture war. I prefer the middle ground where I can see multiple points of view and evaluate them in the light of my values.

Ken and I have different views on the media and how to prepare our girls to interact with the messages they experience through movies and TV that offend our sensibilities. My approach has been to allow them to view most popular content, even if that content is offensive or contrary to our values. But I often participate in the viewing (or listening, in the case of pop music) so we can have meaningful discussions. Ken's approach is different. He prefers to prescreen questionable media or avoid it altogether if he feels ill-prepared to interact with it. He tends to restrict viewing of materials that are offensive or contrary to his values in an effort to communicate a standard to our girls.

While Ken and I agree that we need to set standards, we also know we need to negotiate in the gray areas. For example, Ken tends to be more permissive in allowing our girls to watch violent content, and I tend to be more permissive in allowing them to watch some sexual content. We obviously draw the line at viewing of pornography. In all the gray areas, Ken and I agree that it's important to view questionable content along with our girls so we can guide them in understanding that content in light of our family and faith commitments.

Parents and children experience many conflicts in the midst of evolving relationships, and those conflicts often result in an us versus them world—parent versus teen, husband versus wife, sibling versus sibling, and sometimes even us against the world. Drs. John and Julie Gottman, clinical psychologists and marriage therapists, have studied marital conflict for decades. Their research shows that couples who approach conflict as opponents needing to win a battle often end up losing relationally in the long run. But couples who approach conflict as members of the same team working toward the same goal tend to experience more staying power in their marriages.[1]

There were some shows we did not permit the girls to watch based on Ken's assessment, and there were some we didn't let them watch based on my assessment. Sometimes we agreed; sometimes we didn't. We both participated in screening what our kids were watching, though we didn't always watch every episode with them. We trusted that we would hear about questionable content in conversations around the dinner table or in the car on the way to church or sporting events.

Ken and I share the goal of teaching our daughters to make wise choices and to know right from wrong. We don't always see eye to eye on how to reach that goal, and we're gifted in different ways, so sometimes there is no way to compromise—we just do things differently. And that's okay for our girls. They're different too, so sometimes his approach is most helpful and sometimes mine is.

Looking back I realize I had quite a bit of anxiety in the midst of conversations about homosexuality. I knew a young woman who was disowned by her church and family when she discovered she was attracted to women. She was threatened at her Christian college after the rumors came out, and she has since lost her faith and refuses to go to any church. She's still estranged from her family and faith community. I don't ever want that for my daughters.

I've shared my fears with Ken and we've worked through my anxiety together. His steadfastness and loyalty give me strength and courage when I'm feeling weak. I tend to react by processing my emotions externally in the moment. Ken processes internally and over time. His calm exterior helps me stay grounded when I'm tempted to fly off into the atmosphere of fear.

Fear continues to be a factor in my interactions with my girls. But I am striving to overcome fear and shame.

8

Fear Factor

M y daughter Katie, age sixteen, still wore her purity ring even though it seemed like her relationship with her boyfriend was becoming less "pure" all the time. Her dad was suspicious from the beginning. After all, one of Ken's first experiences with the boy was when he read some text messages on Katie's phone that contained multiple uses of the "F" word. I shrugged it off as normal teenage banter—until I was heading home from one of my weekly Portland trips.

While I was on the train ride home, I got a text from Karen. "Did Dad tell you what happened with Katie?"

"No. What's up?"

"You'll find out when you get home."

The first chance I had to talk with Ken privately after returning home, I asked about Katie. He didn't give me too many details because Katie had asked to tell me herself. But I got the bare minimum—she had been Skyping with her boyfriend using Karen's computer and didn't realize the transcript of the text portion of the conversation was being saved. The next time Karen went on Skype, she discovered the explicit nature of

Katie's conversation with her boyfriend. Katie was busted!

Katie did eventually tell me what had happened. And to some degree, I could relate. I remembered how much I wanted to have sex at her age.

Bonding

A few weeks later, on Mother's Day, I decided to follow up on the Skype incident.

"Katie, I know you really like Paul and want to have sex with him. But I'm worried you're going to make a decision you'll regret." I rolled down the car window as I pulled out of the shopping center parking garage. Critical conversations in the car were my specialty.

"Mom, you don't need to worry about me." She tuned the radio to her favorite station.

"Well, I do worry, especially when I think about all the mistakes I made at your age. I'd like to tell you a few stories about bonding, okay?"

"Okay."

I turned down the radio before launching in.

"I decided to have sex when I was sixteen. And then I had a bunch of casual relationships while I was in college. I had one serious relationship before I met your dad, and we lived together. All of those relationships had a lasting effect on me. Your dad lived with someone too before I met him, so neither of us were virgins when we met. But we decided to wait to have sex with each other until our wedding night. It wasn't easy."

Katie nodded, giving me permission to keep talking.

"One of the hardest things when your dad and I were dating was for me to trust him—to believe that every time he kissed me he wasn't trying to have sex with me. My body remembered all those previous relationships. There were bonds formed in my brain that taught my body how one thing leads to another. But it wasn't just those bonds that remained; there were also emotional bonds connected to feelings of rejection, pain from feeling unloved after a one-night stand, and feelings of regret and fear. Every time your dad would kiss me and try to hold me close, my body would erupt in a confusing mess of mixed emotions. I love your dad and wanted to kiss him a lot! But my body was full of fear. Even after we got married, I struggled. My counselor has helped me heal from some of those things and reconfigure those bonds—but it's been hard work."

"But you and dad are okay. I mean, you have four kids and everything turned out fine."

"I don't know if I'd say everything has always been fine. But, yes, we work through hard things together and survive. My question for you is, do you want Paul to be such a significant part of your story for the rest of your life?"

"I don't know, Mom. I really like him. And it's really hard."

"Katie, I'm telling you these things because I love you very much."

"I know, Mom. If I didn't know you love me, I would have had sex already!"

Reflection. I was amazed at this statement—at how intuitively Katie connected her feelings about being loved by her parents with her feelings about waiting to have sex. Katie and I ended up having many conversations about her Skype incident. She eventually broke up with the guy after he spread rumors about her that weren't true. She was tempted to have "breakup sex" with some random dude, and we talked about that. We discussed her identity development, and we talked about how sex bonds two people in significant, mysterious and complex ways. Some people even argue that having sexual intercourse is marriage in God's eyes.[1]

I carried the complexity of my physical and emotional bonds throughout my life. No matter how hard I tried to have "casual sex" when I was young, there was never anything casual about it. Bonding is real. When we bond with others through sexual intercourse, a part of that person remains with us for the rest of our lives.

A strong parental bond is the factor that has the highest correlation with young people waiting until later for sexual debut. Teens who wait to have sex report close relationships with one or both of their parents. Parental bonding is not a panacea, but it's an important factor in helping our girls make wise choices about who they are, who they will choose to be and with whom they will have sex. Even if they choose to have sex before marriage, a strong parental bond and openness to talking about our girls' decisions without judgment and condemnation can help them make wise choices—even if those choices are not the ones we had hoped for.

If our girls make a choice they later regret, will we be the kind of parents who model grace and peace and help them learn from those choices? We need to balance truth with grace and emphasize our girls' participation in choosing God's will, God's desire, God's intention. This is our desire for them as well, but ultimately it is their choice. Our responsibility is to clearly explain the choice and inspire loyalty to Jesus, not to a set of rules and regulations. It is only relationship with the living God that will empower young people to overcome the powerful temptations of the flesh, the world and the devil. Helping them discover their authentic selves will lead them to encounter the God who created them. If we communicate only how bad, terrible or wrong it is to have sexual intercourse before marriage, we risk losing our girls into a life full of fear and shame. When all they can imagine is the worst-case scenario, they stop imagining and start escaping. Let's help them imagine who they are and who they can be as cooperative participants in God's kingdom, living lives of creative goodness for the sake of others.

True Love Waits for What?

Not long after the True Love Waits abstinence campaign began in 1993, studies on the efficacy of purity pledges started appearing. Unfortunately, these studies rarely agreed with one another. Some suggested that virginity pledges correlated with a delay in sexual debut, while others showed no difference between pledgers and nonpledgers when similar groups of teens were compared. The results of all these studies indicate that abstinence has to come from an individual conviction rather than participation in a program. Factors such as parental attitude toward sex, religious convictions and a teen's perception of her friends' attitudes about sex play more important roles than the pledge itself.

• • •

The secret Katie was keeping welled up into tears.

"Mom, I have something I need to tell you." Katie, seventeen, was wearing her favorite blue sweater that brought out the bright blue in her eyes, but her eyes didn't seem so bright just then.

"Okay. Do you want to talk now?" I set aside the mail I was reading and gave her my full attention.

"Can we go upstairs? It's kind of private." She folded her arms across her chest and waited.

"Sure." I placed the important mail in my respond-to-later pile and the junk mail in the recycle pile so I could pick up where I left off when I came back downstairs.

We went into my room and sat on the end of my bed.

"What's up?" I faced her as she sat with her legs crisscrossed and her hands clenched together in her lap.

"Mom, I had sex." Her lower lip was trembling and I could see a tear begin to spill out of the corner of her eye. But she was good at stopping the flood. Only one managed to escape.

"Okay." I didn't know what to say, so I decided to ask some questions. "When did you have sex and who was it with?"

"It was a while ago and it was with Kevin. You don't know him." She choked back a few more tears and brought her pinky finger up to her mouth to bite her nail.

"Why are you telling me now and why are you so upset?" I reached out and held her other hand, which was still resting in her lap.

"Well, you just got that book contract and I was afraid that what I had done would ruin things for you. That you won't be able to write the book because of me." She hung her head and stared at our clasped hands.

At that moment, my heart broke. And the tears that had been welling up in her eyes came pouring out of mine.

I reached over and wrapped both my arms around her as she rested her head on my shoulder and let the tears she had been holding in seep onto my shirt.

Reflection. My heart didn't break over the fact that Katie had decided to have sex. I wasn't that surprised, actually. After all, she was the one who had been Skyping and talking about sex with her boyfriend the year before. No, my heart broke over the fear and shame she had lived with for months.

Most of the time Katie didn't have the opportunity to keep secrets—somehow, she always got caught. Yet this one thing—

this one really important thing—she managed to keep hidden for months. But she couldn't keep it hidden any longer. Her confession came just days after I received the contract to write this book.

One thing I've wanted to be certain to do as a parent is to distinguish between poor choices, bad behavior and "being bad." My husband and I tried to remind each other not to say things like "bad girl" or "I can't believe you were dumb enough to do that." We tried to correct bad behavior and encourage our girls to make wise choices. We tried not to shame them.

Remember the difference between guilt and shame?

- Guilt = I did something bad/wrong.
- Shame = I *am* bad/wrong.

Guilt is supposed to lead to confession and, when wrong actions are corrected, to transformation and deeper connection with God and others. On the other hand, shame almost certainly leads to hiding wrong behavior for fear of rejection and abandonment and often leads to disconnection from God, others and our true selves. Shame communicates that doing something wrong means there's something fundamentally wrong with the core of who I am.

No matter how hard we try as parents to correct wrong behavior and avoid shaming our children, shame still manages to infect them. We say "That was a bad thing you did" instead of "You are so bad!" We train them to ask for forgiveness and try to teach them to make better choices. Then we say we forgive them. But we keep treating them as if they're going to keep doing that wrong thing. We try to trust them to learn from their mistakes—while we give them the third degree, making them prove their goodness over and over again. Deep inside we know they will make poor choices again. A part of us remembers they are not perfect, but we forget that it's kindness that leads to a change of heart.

I held my precious daughter tight. My heart was breaking not just over her fear of rejection, which made her keep her secret hidden for so many months, but over her fear that her choice might lead others to reject me too. Not only did she imagine that what she had done made her a bad person; she feared it would make me a bad person too. You see, shame is infectious. It spreads like a dragnet, catching many in its trap. It sweeps us in, and before we know it we've been snatched out of the life-giving water of grace and acceptance and dumped onto the hard, dry ground of fear and self-loathing.

· · ·

"Oh, Katie. You don't have to worry about me. It doesn't matter whether I write a book or not. What matters is whether you're okay."

"But we did that purity thing and I failed you." She heaved a few more sobs onto my shoulder.

"Katie, the purity thing isn't about me. I just wanted to help you make wise choices and be safe. Were you safe? Did you use protection?" I released her from my embrace and gave her a tissue to wipe her eyes.

"Yes, of course. I'm not stupid." She wiped at the mascara that had smudged her freckled cheeks.

"Was it breakup sex after Paul?" I reached over and gently wiped a few more streaks of mascara off her cheek.

"Yes, and it wasn't even that good."

"Are you still having sex?" I was curious and wanted more details about her first encounter, wishing it were something worth celebrating.

"No, Mom. I'm not having sex with anyone. The next time I

want it to be with someone I love. I was really upset after Paul broke up with me and felt so rejected. I wanted him to be my first. I thought I was ready and I just wanted to do it. I thought it would make me feel better. It didn't." She started biting her pinky again so I grabbed her hands and held them tightly as I sat cross-legged with my knees touching hers.

"Katie, no matter what, I want you to know that I love you very much. I'm not mad at you. I'm just sad that your first time wasn't a sweet memory for you. I'm sad it wasn't with someone you love."

"I know. Me too."

I held her close again and told her how much I loved her. I assured her that she had not ruined my reputation. I reminded her that she was not defined by her mistakes.

I am still amazed by the courage Katie showed that day. In the face of paralyzing fear, she opened her heart and let me see her cry. She shared her pain and fear of rejection. She confessed that she felt like she had failed me and failed herself. I held her tender heart in my hands as she melted in my arms one more time.

"We need to tell your dad," I whispered in her ear. "Do you want to do it by yourself or do you want to do it with me?"

She leaned back out of my embrace and quickly replied, "With you. I want you to be there."

"Well, your dad is home, so I'll go get him and we can tell him together." I left her sitting there with the tissue box close at hand.

Ken joined us on the bed. Katie was sitting at the bottom corner on his side. He sat up near his pillow and I sat next to her on the end. Katie told him about her first time having sex. He asked for a few details to understand how she'd snuck around to get away with it. After a few moments of going over the particulars, he gave her a big hug and told her how much he loved her.

We embraced her together and offered to pray for her. We prayed that she would know how much she was loved. We asked God to help her know that she was valuable. We begged God to be present with her in a way that would allow her to experience the love of Christ and the power of the Holy Spirit in tangible ways. We expressed our confidence that she would learn from her mistakes. We trusted God with her future choices and prayed that she would not let others define her by her mistakes. We said "Amen" as we all agreed that nothing could separate us from the love of God and from the love of one another.

Some of the youth at church knew the trouble Katie had gotten herself into—the things she had been caught doing, the rumors that swirled around her. It was hard for her to go to church knowing they knew those things, knowing they might sit in judgment and talk about her behind her back. Some Sundays she felt the condemning glances more than others, but she kept showing up and opening up her heart to those she trusted to keep on loving her and accepting her no matter what. Some days she felt like she didn't really fit in. Was she even worthy of being called a Christian after all the mistakes she had made?

She felt a bit of subtle shunning and shaming that troubled her heart. She was rarely invited to be part of the events for students who were "on fire" for Jesus. Some assumed she didn't care about Jesus as much as others. She wasn't the type to talk about her faith all the time. But Jesus was as real to her as to anyone else. Maybe even more real. Katie knows about grace. She knows about unconditional love. While some are standing around raising stones of condemnation, she hears Jesus calling her "daughter." She hears Jesus inviting her to go and sin no more. She hears Jesus and answers, with a cry from deep within her heart, "yes, I will go."

It's hard to shake the labels of shame—sinner, heathen, failure, troubled teen, rebellious, uncommitted, unfaithful, worldly, materialistic, selfish, hypocrite, lost, out of control. Those are just a few of the labels that get thrown around in some Christian churches—places where people are supposed to be full of grace, bringers of hope, bearers of good news, lovers of one another. It takes courage to share your heart not knowing whether grace will be offered or shame will be smeared.

We scheduled a time to talk with Katie's youth leader, Neely. Katie asked me to be there with her. Neely was not surprised. She had heard the rumors. Neely had been Katie's leader for years and heard other confessions at youth camps and small group meetings that I was not aware of. That's why I trusted Neely. Neely prayed with Katie and embraced her with kindness and grace. Kindness changes things. Grace makes a difference.

My daughter has shown courage in her willingness to be vulnerable. She keeps opening her heart to me and to her friends and has found power in her vulnerability. She agreed to let me tell this story, hoping it would help parents and others extend kindness and grace to young Christian women who don't live up to the ideals of purity culture.

She stands stronger today because she had the courage to confess, to let me and others see her failures and listen to her heart cry when she needed to know she was worthy of love even in the midst of deep sorrow and regret. She may have made some bad choices, but haven't we all?

Brené Brown defines vulnerability not as weakness but as courage, emotional risk, exposure and uncertainty. Katie took a risk in sharing her secret with me. She couldn't predict what my response would be, but she faced the uncertainty and opened up anyway. Shame is a powerful enemy. Shame is fueled by secrecy, silence and judgment. Shame is healed by vulnerability, self-compassion, compassion from others and empathy.[2] Together, we were able to defeat the enemy of shame.

When we worry about the sexual choices our girls might make during their teen years, what are our worst fears? Are we afraid we will lose our reputation as parents or leaders in our faith communities? Are we afraid we will be shamed by our girls? Are we afraid their future will be ruined and they will never be able to recover from their bad decisions? Do we fear they will keep making bad choices and eventually go off the deep end? Whatever our fears, it's important to name them, to confess them and to find the courage to face them and come out the other side.

One of my own great fears is that I have done harm to my girls and that I have shamed them and made them feel un-lovable and unworthy of my love. While I try hard to communicate the difference between guilt and shame, I am not perfect. And sometimes shame still makes its way through.

Fear and shame are powerful allies. If we want to avoid shaming others, we have to overcome our own fears. Fear feeds shame. Faith starves shame. As Paul reminds us in Romans 10:11, "Anyone who believes in him will never be put to shame." Will we choose to believe in the kind of love who died for us while we were yet sinners? Will we show that kind of love to our daughters? Will we tell them, while you are not yet perfect, while you are not quite as pure as I imagined you were, I will love you? Will we remember that we are yet sinners too?

Here's a prayer and a poem I offered my daughter after her courageous confession.

> Dear daughter, I love you and always will. I love your courage to be honest with me no matter what fears may be tempting you to hide in shame. I love the beauty of your deepest heart cry, your longing to love and be loved, your hope to find grace and peace in a world filled with shame and fear. I love your passion to help deliver others from the power of shame and systems of oppression. I love the way you offer grace to others and refuse to pick up stones of condemnation. I love the way you stand strong and offer strength to others when they are feeling weakened by shame and fear.

#facingthetalk: Don't let anxiety and fear over what might happen ruin your relationship with your daughter. Be realistic—girls *are* doing it. Talk honestly and openly about your concerns and practice empathy. Trust that your kindness will help them make wise choices in the future.

She's a Big Girl Now

"Karen, you need to get out of bed. You can't sleep all day."

Only grumbling sounds emerged from the bed.

"Karen, I'm not joking. You need to get up and come to dinner and do your homework."

She rolled over and pulled the blanket over her head—which sent me into lecture mode.

"It's not healthy for you to stay in bed all day. You need to get involved in some kind of sport or get a job after school. And you need to eat regular meals. Eating healthy meals at regular times helps you have energy. Is there something else going on at school that I need to know about? Are you feeling depressed?"

"Mom, stop! I'm just tired. Leave me alone!"

"Karen, I'm your mom. I'm not going to leave you alone. Your health is important to me and I'm worried about you. You need to get out of bed and come to dinner."

The power struggle had begun.

"I'm not hungry. Now go away!"

"I'll leave your room as soon as you get out of bed."

"Mom! Leave me alone. I don't feel good."

I left the room exasperated, afraid if I stayed I would say something I would regret. I went to the kitchen and asked Ken when dinner would be ready. Fifteen minutes. By then a little bit of wisdom had bubbled up. I asked him to help.

"Karen isn't listening to me and we're stuck in a power struggle. Will you go ask her to come to dinner? Sometimes I'm just not good at giving her choices."

"Okay, I'll go talk to her. Will you stir the cheese sauce?"

I traded places with him at the stove and stirred the cheese sauce for his famous homemade macaroni and cheese. It was my grandma's recipe, but he had modified it and improved on it over the years. It was now a Chapin family specialty.

Ken knocked on Karen's bedroom door.

"Karen, dinner will be ready in about ten minutes. Do you want me to come in and drag you out of bed, or do you want to get up by yourself?"

Ken's approach to giving choices was a little different from mine.

"No, don't come in! I'll get up myself."

Ken returned to the kitchen just in time to drain the noodles and combine them with the cheese. I went to gather the rest of the girls for dinner.

This scenario repeated itself over the next few weeks before I started asking more questions.

This time I sat on the edge of her bed calmly.

"Karen, you seem really tired lately. Are you on your period?"

"Yes, I've been bleeding for a while now." She faced the wall and mumbled into her pillow.

"How long is a while?"

"I don't know. Maybe a couple of weeks."

"Why didn't you tell me? That's not normal."

"I didn't know. They said periods would be irregular for a while when you're a teenager. I just thought this was part of being irregular." She rolled over to face me. Her fair skin masked the pallor in her cheeks.

"We need to get you in to see a doctor as soon as possible. It's almost time for your annual physical anyway. I'm so sorry you haven't been feeling well."

"Mom, I can barely walk home from school without falling asleep on the way. I'm so exhausted. I fell asleep babysitting for just a minute the other day and the mom freaked out. It's frustrating. You and Dad just think I'm being lazy and irresponsible, but I'm not. I just don't feel good."

"I'm sorry I've been so hard on you. We will figure this out together. I'll make an appointment for the doctor tomorrow." I reached over to stroke her arm and she let me.

Reflection. Fear and shame can sometimes blind us to what's really going on. I was afraid that I had done something to cause Karen to stop participating in sports and gain weight. I was ashamed of some of the ways I had disciplined her when she was younger and feared that my failure as a parent had caused her pain—that her weight gain was a symptom of emotional issues that were my fault. My fear and shame prevented me from paying attention to other important factors that were present in her life.

We went to the doctor together and discovered that Karen had a hormonal imbalance that likely caused not only weight gain but anemia. No wonder she was tired all the time. But discovering this physical issue didn't help me overcome my fear and shame completely. To this day I still struggle with feeling like it was somehow my fault. I also struggle with fear that this hormonal imbalance will lead to more serious problems. We've tried natural hormone treatments, and now that Karen is an adult she has tried using birth control to manage her periods. It's been a struggle.

Ten days after Karen turned eighteen, she ended up in the emergency room with a serious condition that the doctors could not explain. My first question was whether it was hormone-related. The doctors told me it was likely unrelated to hormones and described the condition as idiopathic—arising spontaneously or without a known cause.

Still, I think it's possible that Karen's hormone imbalances could have contributed to the onset of this issue. Hormonal imbalances contribute to many health concerns in girls and women—far more than just PMS. When I was in my early twenties I was diagnosed with endometriosis, uterine fibroids and a tumor on my left ovary. I had surgery to remove my ovary and the fibroids and to take care of the endometriosis. I continue to have fears for my daughters about their health. Hormonal imbalances don't just impact our reproductive health; they can affect mental health, emotional health and physical health as well. While we shouldn't blame all moodiness on PMS—

sometimes young women are grumpy because they're tired or hurt—we should be aware of the symptoms.

There were many times I became fearful as my girls continued to mature and encounter more challenges in life. Sometimes the fears were connected with hurts from my past, other times they were related to the very real and present dangers we encounter every day. I had to learn to face my fears, and sometimes I needed help facing those fears. My mentors and counselors were invaluable resources in helping me heal from my past hurts and find strategies to respond to dangerous situations my daughters might encounter at school, when hanging out with friends or through interactions with others online. When my daughters had health concerns, I not only consulted trusted medical advisers but had close friends who walked with us as we faced those challenges. It is important to face your fears and seek help when you feel as if your fears are overwhelming you. It is possible to overcome fears, but in order to overcome them we first have to face them.

9

Overcoming Fear and Shame

*T*een dramas, movies, social media and peers are constantly presenting our girls with the message that their value is in their beauty or sex appeal. They are invited into exciting stories of risk-taking and pleasure-seeking through sexual exploits, drugs, cutting and other harmful behaviors. The alternative offered to many Christian girls is a story born out of fear—an invitation to stay safe and to protect themselves from the evils of the world. This subtly implies that pleasure is bad and God doesn't take risks—so neither should we. God's story of passionate pursuit of his people and willingness to take risks to show love is often overlooked and neglected when we focus on keeping our girls safe.

I intended to take my girls on one last trip before they went off to college to experience being on a team to serve others, but many overseas opportunities were not only expensive; they were risky. While I wanted to invite them to join God's work in the world, how much of a risk was I willing to take?

Letting Go

This time Karen wasn't trapped in the car. At age eighteen, she'd joined me on the road trip willingly. Actually, the road trip had been her idea. I was the one who was nervous this time.

A month before this last getaway, we'd had quite an argument.

"Mom, it's not fair. You promised you would take me on another getaway before college. When and where are we going? Summer is almost over!" Karen threw a few more T-shirts in the giveaway pile as she sorted through the clothes she'd need for college.

"I know. I'm sorry things haven't worked out like we'd hoped. The service trips organized through the church are just too expensive and I haven't had time to do any fundraising." I grabbed a shirt from the giveaway pile and tried to convince her to keep it. It was one of my favorites on her.

"Mom, I don't like that shirt. You don't know me or understand me anymore. You say you care and that you want to do this special trip with me, but you're too busy to plan it and make it happen. I wish you'd never promised. It just makes me mad." She grabbed the shirt from me and threw it back in the giveaway pile.

"Well, you could do some research and planning too. You know, you're an adult now. You don't need me to do everything for you. Why don't *you* figure out where we should go?"

"I don't know how to figure it out. I don't know how much money we can spend or where we could stay. And I'm not good at organizing things—just look at my room!"

Her room was a mess. It was often a mess.

"Well, my room is a mess too and I have papers to grade and I still have to plan Kimberly's second trip. I'm not neglecting you; it's just been busy with both of us graduating and me starting a new job and you getting ready to go to college," I said. "I want to take you on another getaway—I'm just not sure how to make it work." I frowned over another favorite shirt getting thrown into the giveaway pile.

"Whatever."

"I'm not going to make any promises, but I'm still trying to figure something out. If you have any ideas, let me know."

The next week Karen ran into a friend from church who was heading to Mexico to work in an orphanage for a few months teaching English. Before she knew it, she had a plan.

"Mom, can we take a road trip to Mexico and visit my friend at the orphanage for my getaway? Please?" She put on her brightest "I know you really love me" smile.

"I don't know. Is there a place for us to stay there? What about the problems at the border? How much is it going to cost? What do you know about the orphanage?"

"Mackenzie says there's room for us to stay with her and I'll help pay for gas. We can stay with Nana on our way down, and don't you have friends in San Diego we could stay with?" She answered all my questions about the orphanage, but I was still concerned about the border conflicts.

"I'm not sure. You figure out how much it will cost to drive down there and I'll check into who we could stay with in San Diego. I also need to know more about how risky it is to cross the border right now."

We worked out the details in the next few weeks. I really didn't feel safe driving across the border and it was too expensive to get the extra insurance. So Karen made plans with her friend to pick us up and take us across the border.

We spent a few days serving at the orphanage and Karen fell in love with many of the children there. She didn't want to leave. But school started in a few days, so we left Mexico and began the long drive back to Seattle.

"Mom, can we adopt Pablo and his little brothers?"

"I don't think so. You have three sisters. Where would we put them all?"

"They can have my room. I'll be at school. Please, Mom? They shouldn't have to live at the orphanage. Pablo is too old; nobody's going to adopt him. And I don't want him to be separated from his brothers. It's just not right." She folded her arms and stared out the window. I think she had tears in her eyes.

"I know it's not right but adopting is a big responsibility. We can talk to your dad about it when we get home, but don't get your hopes up. Maybe you can adopt when you're older. You are very compassionate and caring and I'm sure you'll get a chance to help somehow."

"It's just terrible that their parents don't want them. I heard the mom keeps getting arrested for doing drugs and the dad is really violent. They need someone to love them! I really want to adopt them. Alejandro, the youngest one, is so sweet!"

"Karen, do you understand why those kids are in the orphanage?"

"I heard some of the stories. I guess their parents just don't want them."

"It's probably more complicated than that. Sometimes people have children and can't take care of them. Maybe they aren't old enough to properly care for them or they don't have enough money. Sometimes children are taken away from parents because of drugs or violence, like Pablo and his brother." I had planned to talk with her about relationship violence, and this seemed like the right opportunity.

"It makes me so mad. I can't believe parents could actually hurt their children!"

"I know. It's hard to believe. Child abuse and domestic violence are really complicated. I've told you a little bit about my story growing up, but I think it might be time for you to know some more of the details. It's important for you to know some of our family history so you can be aware of potential problems that might come up for you."

I told her some of the details of my childhood experiences with domestic violence and sexual abuse. It was hard.

"Karen, I know it makes you sad to think about these things. But if you ever want to ask me questions about it or talk with me about it more, just let me know."

"Mom, that sounds like it was terrible. It makes me sad and it's hard to believe Grandpa would do that stuff to Nana. I'm glad he eventually got help for his problems. I don't have any questions right now and I don't really want to talk about it anymore. It makes me mad. Can we just listen to music for a while? I'm tired." She put her feet up on the dash and put her pillow up against the window to settle in for a nap.

Reflection. I had talked with Karen in general about domestic violence and sexual abuse over the years, but I waited until she was an adult before telling any specific details about my story. My father passed away in 2006, and many years before that my sister and I had talked with him about his past abuse. While it was still a private and personal topic, it wasn't a family secret. Once girls are adults, there are many topics that are helpful to discuss as they encounter more issues in the world around them.

For me, talking about violence and sexual assault was important. I was fortunate that my daughters never got into any violent relationships, but teen-dating violence is an important topic to think about and touch on periodically. My daughters have had friends who experienced teen-dating violence and sexual assault. Recently, Katie asked for my advice on how to help a friend in a potentially dangerous situation. Together we came up with a plan that we hoped would lead to her getting help.

In many ways, my goal for the sex talk getaways has been accomplished—I have good relationships with my daughters and they're not afraid to talk to me about sex. They're not always comfortable talking about it, but for the most part they're not afraid. They also know they have access to many other resources. If they don't want to talk with me, they can talk to their youth leader or another trusted adult.

Many people face fear and experience shame in talking with their children about sex. The roots of my own fear and shame were in my experiences of trauma and abuse. For others, fear and shame might be rooted in silence. Still others may have grown up in a culture that taught that sex was dirty and once they got married they had a hard time overcoming those negative messages. We are just now starting to see the effects of purity culture. While some religious couples who wait until marriage to participate in sexual intercourse have good experiences after marriage, others do not. Tina Schermer Sellers, a certified sex therapist, works with clients who struggle with religious sexual shame.[1] We each have a unique story that influences how we talk to our daughters about sex. Hopefully, my story has inspired you to think about your own story as you journey with your daughters and talk about sex.

I wish I could promise that your daughter will choose to live into a better story than the one the world offers after you find healing in your own story, talk honestly about sex and go on getaways with her. Well, I can't promise, but I do have hope. I have hope for the future. I believe an emerging generation of young women and men committed to being cooperative friends of Jesus is arising. And we can help them. We can help them set things right in the world.

We can encourage them to live lives of creative goodness in

the power of the Holy Spirit for the sake of others. We can model for them a love of God that invites them into cooperative relationship with Jesus. These things we can do.

Without a doubt, our children will make some mistakes during their teen and young adult years. And it won't do them any good if we try to prevent those mistakes by making their choices for them. After all, how can we expect them to make wise choices if we don't ever let them choose how they want to live? How can they learn to make things right if they never make any mistakes? Some wise teachers taught me to let our children make mistakes while the cost is low. This is especially hard to do in the area of sexuality if we fear that they will live a life of regret over any mistakes they make and that those mistakes will ruin them forever.

One of my favorite movie quotes about regret is from *13 Going on 30*. At age thirteen, Jenna Rink makes a decision to align herself with a certain group of kids, rejecting her childhood best friend in the process. She is then magically given the opportunity to see what that choice would lead to by becoming her thirteen-year-old self trapped in her future thirty-year-old body. After a while, she realizes she doesn't like the thirty-year-old she has become. She goes home to try to figure things out and asks her mom about regrets.

"Well, Jenna, I know I made a lot of mistakes, but I don't regret making any of them," Beverly Rink says.

"How come?" Jenna asks.

Beverly replies, "Because if I hadn't made them, I wouldn't have learned how to make things right."

We have to let our girls make mistakes. But we also have to teach them how to make things right. One of the ways we can do this is by making things right in our own story. Of course, we still want to teach them how to make wise choices in the first place. What if we communicated our trust in their ability to make wise choices in the area of sexuality like this:

- We believe God's intention for sex is to facilitate long-term bonding, deep intimacy and shared pleasure.

- When you are a teenager, it's more risky to bond and more difficult to find deep intimacy.

- If you choose to experiment with bonding, intimacy and pleasure in sexual relationships before marriage, we will still love you.

- We trust you will make wise choices about protecting yourself from unwanted pregnancy and sexually transmitted diseases. If that means waiting until you are older and married, we will celebrate that choice with you.

- If you make a mistake and have unprotected sex and get pregnant or get an STD, we will love you and be with you as you figure out what to do.

- No matter what choices you make, we will always love you and celebrate your presence in our lives.

If empathy is the enemy of shame, we need to remember our stories. Instead of trying to guide our girls with rules and regulations, let's be with them in relationship and offer narratives of grace and truth.

After all, isn't the incarnation about empathy? Empathy is the ability to understand and share the feelings of another. The writer of Hebrews says of Jesus, "For we do not have a high priest who is unable to empathize with our weaknesses, but we have one who has been tempted in every way, just as we are—yet he did not sin" (Hebrews 4:15). That last bit, "yet he did not sin," is not there to shame us—if Jesus could avoid temptation then I should too, so if I can't there must be something wrong with me. Nor is it there to give us an excuse to sin—Jesus is God, of course he didn't sin, but you can't expect that of me; I'm only human and I'll never be anything more than a failure.

Here's what that verse is saying: once we believe in Jesus, we don't ever have to be ashamed of being human. But we still struggle with shame. One of the most important aspects of being human is knowing we are not God. That's why a confession of faith is so important. When we confess our faith we acknowledge before God and others that we are not God—Jesus is. The only human who could ever truly know right from wrong and do it is Jesus. And Jesus invites us into the greatest story of all.

Jesus invites us into a story that says the only way to be appropriately connected with God and others is to allow ourselves to be shaped and formed by the one who made us, the one who wants to be with us, the one who loves us and accepts us even in our deepest shame.

If you have fear and shame that you need to overcome in your own story, I invite you to begin to practice the following simple disciplines.

1. Confess your failures, hurts and struggles to God and ask God what truth the Spirit wants to say to you about who you are in light of that confession. Take time to listen. Memorize verses about your identity in Christ to help you hear God's truth more clearly.

2. Speak truth to yourself in the form of a paradox prayer. Catherine Skurja in *Paradox Lost* helped me understand that in order to uncover my true identity in Christ, I had to acknowledge the things I was most ashamed of.[2] Paradox prayers

have helped me to overcome fear and shame. Take the thing you feel shame about and put it in the first part of the prayer. Shame is usually associated with the failures, hurts and struggles that we need to confess. The prayer goes like this:

Even though I am _____, I am loved and accepted by God. (Insert the source of your shame, failure, hurt or struggle in the space provided.)

Here are some of my paradox prayers:

- *Even though I had sex for the first time before I got married, I am loved and accepted by God.*

- *Even though I get angry and yell at my girls sometimes, I am loved and accepted by God.*

- *Even though I was abused as a child, I am loved and accepted by God.*

These are just simple guides to get you started. I highly recommend seeking help to overcome shame from your past and find healing from wrongs done to you. Whether you get help through a recovery program, group counseling or individual sessions with a therapist, trained counselor or spiritual director, you will not regret it.

Isn't such paradoxical love and acceptance the heart of the gospel message? God relentlessly pursued Israel even when she repeated her mistakes and chose death instead of life. Jesus came and died so we would know the full extent of God's love. Romans 5:8 says, "But God demonstrates his own love for us in this: While we were still sinners, Christ died for us." And Jesus rose from the dead to bring us closer to God's heart, to bring us into the full embrace of the Trinity.

How will we demonstrate God's love to our girls? Will we

shame them and reject them when they don't live up to our righteous purity standards? Or will we embrace them and do as Christ commanded: love one another?

I've continued to have sex talks with my girls even after they turned eighteen. I could narrate a few more interesting stories for you, but it's their turn to start writing their own stories.

One thing I keep reminding them of during this transitional phase into independent adulthood is that I will love them no matter where they live. And I will love them no matter whom they choose to love. There is nothing they can do to stop me from loving them.

Acknowledgments

irst, I must acknowledge that writing a book, especially one that is largely memoir, is harder than I ever imagined. Without the inspiration and encouragement of many, I never would have been able to do the hard work required to produce this manuscript. I would first like to acknowledge the editors who rejected my first book proposal, but encouraged me to keep writing. I have dreamed of writing a book since I was a young adult, and it's been a joy to live into that dream.

I'm grateful for the many women in my life who asked me to write this book after hearing of the many conversations I had with my daughters about sex, especially Anne Alecci, who not only insisted that I write this book but listened to and read many early versions of the manuscript. Her advocacy for women who have experienced unplanned pregnancies continues to inspire my work.

I am deeply and significantly indebted to my writing coach, Kimberly George. Without her gracious and spacious guidance I never would have been able to do the intellectual and emotional work necessary to write these stories. Her excellent coaching has also influenced the course of my future.

MaryKate Morse was instrumental in getting me connected with my brilliant editor, Cindy Bunch, whose patient direction helped me move this work from an idea to a work that I hope inspires and encourages many mothers. MaryKate's mentorship has helped me to achieve many vocational goals. Darla Samuelson has also been a critical confidant who listened to me process my own trauma and offered me safe space to get away and do some of my writing.

I am thankful for Sarah Keough and Tiffany Kerns as early readers of the manuscript for their valuable feedback. I'm indebted to Sarah Warnock-Farrand and her help with understanding the original Greek of some New Testament passages about purity. Shannon West, a therapist for teen girls and young women, and Neely McQueen helped me understand today's girl culture, and Tina Schermer-Sellers helped me think deeply about religious sexual shame.

Tara Rigby and Amy Sabado, two of my closest friends, have upheld me and walked closely with me not only in the writing of this book, but also in my parenting. Their contribution to this work should not be underestimated.

My sister, Lori King, was not only an early reader but lived many of these stories with me. Her willingness to tell her story of abuse publicly over the years inspires me and encouraged me to wrestle with the implications of abuse in my parenting and its influence on my conversations with my daughters about sex. We continue to heal together and one day we will be old ladies sitting in rocking chairs on a porch together and we will still be laughing at the days to come.

My mother, Barbara Wood, taught me about forgiveness and perseverance. Her faith and courage have helped me imagine myself as a writer and helped me see this project through to the end when I wanted to give up. Whenever I struggled with how hard it was to do this work, I remembered my mother as a survivor of abuse and pressed on in hopes of preventing what happened to us from happening to others.

There were a few men who supported me on this journey that are worthy of noting. Dan Kimball encouraged me in my pursuit of theological education, which inspired my wrestling with issues of sex and Christianity. Tony Kriz always knows how to ask the hard questions and his friendship gives me hope that men and women really can be just friends. Jim Henderson coached me through the early phases of the concept development for this book and continues to tease me for talking about sex all the time. I'm sure this book will give me opportunities to continue to live into that reality.

Without a doubt, there are many others with whom I have spoken who have challenged my thinking, informed my theology, affirmed my calling and given me a touch of grace. To all who have not been named, I thank you.

Karen, Katie, Kelly and Kimberly—this book would not even exist without you. It would fill up the pages of another entire book for me to adequately acknowledge the ways you have shaped and formed me through your presence in my life. I love you all more than you will ever know, and I will never stop reminding you of your conception stories.

My husband, Ken, has been my solid rock providing stable ground from which I can venture out into new worlds and new experiences. He supported me when I faced the trauma of my past and constantly makes space for me to work through my emotions. He brings the calm to my storms. Ken, I love the way you have participated in some of these conversations with our daughters even though it has felt awkward at times. You continue to faithfully encourage my work and you are the most loyal partner and kind father I could have ever hoped for.

Many counselors, both professional and lay, have helped me heal and find strength to imagine a different world for my daughters. Through all these people and through personal encounters with God, I have experienced the help of the Trinity: my Abba—Father God, my Prince of Peace—Jesus Christ and my Wisest Counselor of all—the Holy Spirit.

Appendix A

Resources for The Talks

*H*ere are some resources you may choose to use in preparation for conversations with your girls. I have organized the resources by age and topic. At different stages of your parenting, you may find you have more time to read than others, so please don't let this list overwhelm you. I encourage you to read a variety of resources and to discuss your family values openly. I didn't find many resources that fit perfectly with our own family's value system, nor have I included all the topics I thought were important. We are complex human beings living in an increasingly complex world. There are many different views on any topic out there, and sex education is no exception. The items on this list range from simple resources on sexual development to academic and theological resources on gender and sexuality. I have separated out the resources on abuse in a separate appendix.

I have not included many links to websites since those links often change, but I do offer a few online resources and encourage you to do your own Internet searches on key issues that are unique to your situation. Trust me, if you or your daughter have experienced it, someone has probably written a blog about it. I hope you will find resources here that fit your social situation and help you communicate your family values.

Books for Preteens and Early Teens

Gitchel, Sam, and Lorri Foster. *Let's Talk About S-E-X: A Guide for Kids 9 to 12 and Their Parents.* Excelsior, MN: Book Peddlers, 2005.

This book is accessible to preteens and teens. It is not written from a Christian perspective but is helpful in covering topics other books might avoid. This book addresses information your daughter might encounter in school health classes that you might not think to talk about. It opens the door for conversations about your family values that may be in contrast to others'.

Graver, Jane, and Len Ebert. *How You Are Changing: For Girls Ages 10-12 and Parents.* Learning About Sex for the Christian Family. St. Louis: Concordia Publishing House, 2008.

I used this book with my girls because it opens with the goodness of God's creation and the goodness of our bodies and sex. The conversation sections are a bit contrived, but overall it offers helpful insights for girls from a Christian perspective.

Hummel, Ruth, and Janet McDonnell. *Where Do Babies Come From? For Girls Ages 7-9.* Learning About Sex for the Christian Family. St. Louis: Concordia Publishing House, 2008.

This is an earlier book in the series I used with my girls. It's a good resource for starting these conversations early.

Madison, Lynda. *The Feelings Book: The Care and Keeping of Your Emotions.* Middleton, WI: American Girl Publishing, 2013.

I wish I had used this book with my oldest daughter but was not familiar with it at the time. This book is helpful in explaining emotional changes and encourages girls to develop strategies so they don't let their emotions control them but rather take control of their own responses to changing emotions.

Metzger, Julie, and Rob Lehman. *Will Puberty Last My Whole Life?* Seattle, WA: Sasquatch Books, 2012.

This book includes real questions from preteens and teens. It is not written from a Christian perspective and includes information for both boys and girls. This book is useful in thinking about the types of conversations your child might be having with peers, or questions your child might be thinking about but is afraid to ask.

Natterson, Cara. *The Care and Keeping of You 2: The Body Book for Older Girls.* Middleton, WI: American Girl Publishing, 2013.

If your preteen is still interested in the American Girl series as she gets older, this updated book for girls ages ten and up offers more details on periods and personal care.

Schaefer, Valorie. *The Care and Keeping of You: The Body Book for Younger Girls.* Middleton, WI: American Girl Publishing, 2012.

This was one of my favorite books. My girls read this on their own and with each other. It was always funny to hear them talking about what stage they thought their younger sister was in as she developed breasts using the stages described in this book. This book is especially good for girls who are interested in the American Girl book series.

Books for Older Teens and Young Adults

Bell, Rob. *Sex God: Exploring the Endless Connections Between Sexuality and Spirituality*. New York: HarperOne, 2012.

Our church youth group used some Rob Bell *Nooma* videos in their services. One of my daughters didn't like his teaching style, but the content of this book helped her frame questions about sex and spirituality as she matured. What I like most about this book is the way it deals with sexual objectification. It also makes some interesting theological concepts accessible for older teens.

Brennan, Dan J. *Sacred Unions, Sacred Passions: Engaging the Mystery of Friendship Between Men and Women*. Elgin, IL: Faith Dance Publishing, 2010.

This book does a great job of disturbing the idea that men and women can't be friends and are destined only to end up in a sexual or romantic relationship.

Godsey, Heather, and Lara Blackwood Pickrel, eds. *Oh God, Oh God, Oh God! Young Adults Speak Out About Sexuality and Christianity*. St. Louis: Chalice Press, 2010.

This collection of essays offers a variety of perspectives from young adult Christians who are involved as leaders or who work for their church. The essay authors come from a wide range of social and theological perspectives and address a broad spectrum of issues from purity to infertility to embodiment and infidelity. Some of these essays are raw and expose the complexity of how young people are wrestling with issues of faith and sexuality today.

Peterson, Margaret Kim, and Dwight N. Peterson. *Are You Waiting for "The One"? Cultivating Realistic, Positive Expectations for Christian Marriage.* Downers Grove, IL: InterVarsity Press, 2011.

This book offers an interesting critique of fairy-tale romantic ideals. My only concern is that it sets up Christian marriage as a new ideal. Overall it offers helpful advice on setting realistic expectations for romantic relationships for those who imagine getting married as an important part of their future.

Books on Parenting

Brown, Brené. *Daring Greatly: How the Courage to Be Vulnerable Transforms the Way We Live, Love, Parent, and Lead.* New York: Gotham Books, 2012.

It is inevitable that at some point your daughter will ask about your first kiss or whether you and your spouse had sex before marriage. Brené Brown is inspirational and offers sound advice for being vulnerable in parenting as well as other aspects of our life.

Burns, Jim. *Teaching Your Children Healthy Sexuality: A Biblical Approach to Prepare Them for Life.* Pure Foundations for Parents. Bloomington, MN: Bethany House, 2008.

This book is available with an accompanying set of CDs or DVDs that can be used in group study. Jim Burns brings

in a variety of experts to discuss relevant topics. I used this
book and the CDs with my youngest daughter. It opened
up the door to many conversations and offers a Christian
perspective on social and sexual issues of our times.

Clark, Chap. *Hurt 2.0: Inside the World of Today's Teenagers.* Grand
Rapids: Baker Academic, 2011.

I have attended a few seminars led by Chap Clark. His
research helps parents and those working with youth understand youth culture today. I recommend this book to
help parents understand that being a teenager today is
vastly different from when they were a teenager.

Cline, Foster, and Jim Fay. *Parenting with Love and Logic: Teaching
Children Responsibility.* Colorado Springs, CO: NavPress, 2006.

This book is foundational for conversations about sexual
health, modesty and beauty standards, as well as dealing with
changing relationships as our children mature into adults.
My favorite aspects of this book are the strategies for mini-
mizing power struggles and for empowering our children to
make wise and responsible decisions. All of this is important
in talking with them about how to be responsible for their
bodies and to set healthy boundaries for themselves.

Haffner, Debra. *From Diapers to Dating: A Parent's Guide to Raising
Sexually Healthy Children.* New York: Newmarket Press, 2008.

This book is my favorite whole-life approach to family-
based sex education. Haffner does not write from a
Christian perspective but offers sound advice for parents
from a variety of faith perspectives. Even if you are starting

later than the diaper years, this book is an important resource to help you think about the ways you have already been talking about sex with your daughter and how you might want to make any adjustments.

Kilbourne, Jean, and Diane E. Levin. *So Sexy So Soon: The New Sexualized Childhood, and What Parents Can Do to Protect Their Kids.* New York: Ballantine Books, 2008.

Church leaders often talk about our oversexualized youth culture. This book offers research to back up such claims as well as strategies for parents to connect with their children and respond to the changing cultural environment.

McMinn, Lisa Graham. *Growing Strong Daughters: Encouraging Girls to Become All They're Meant to Be.* Grand Rapids: Baker Books, 2007.

This book changed my life. It offers helpful sociological research on how girls and women are treated in society as well as an interaction with Christian ethics that helps parents raise their girls to be confident and courageous women in the world today.

Schwartz, Pepper, and Dominic Cappello. *Ten Talks Parents Must Have with Their Children About Sex and Character.* New York: Hachette Books, 2000.

I used this book as inspiration for ways to connect conversations about sex with broader issues of developing character. The scripted conversations are hokey, but the topics are useful.

Wilson, Sandra D. *Released from Shame: Moving Beyond the Pain of the Past.* Downers Grove, IL: InterVarsity Press, 2002.

I found this book helpful as I worked through healing from some of the pain of my past. Even if you haven't experienced trauma growing up, this book will help you identify shame-based family systems and will help you be a grace-filled parent.

Books on Women's Health and Sexuality

Eckert, Kim Gaines. *Things Your Mother Never Told You: A Woman's Guide to Sexuality.* Downers Grove, IL: InterVarsity Press, 2014.

I give this book to my older daughters as a graduation gift. No matter how many conversations we have with our girls about sex, we will never answer all their questions or dispel all the myths they encounter. This book is a must-read for parents and for adult daughters to help keep the conversations going—not just between mother and daughter but with peers as well.

Northrup, Christiane. *Women's Bodies, Women's Wisdom: Creating Physical and Emotional Health and Healing.* New York: Bantam Books, 2010.

This book is a go-to source for many women who have not been taught much about their bodies. Northrup includes wisdom from Eastern traditions as well as Western medicine. This book may be a challenging read for those who have been taught that their passions and sexuality are bad but offers a breadth of knowledge and depth of insight that is hard to find in any other single volume.

Book on Sexuality and Marriage

Leman, Kevin. *Sheet Music: Uncovering the Secrets of Sexual Intimacy in Marriage*. Carol Stream, IL: Tyndale House, 2003.

Writing with Christians in mind, Leman offers forthright yet humorous advice on both physical and emotional intimacy for married couples.

Books on Homosexuality

Hirsch, Debra. *Redeeming Sex: Naked Conversations About Sexuality and Spirituality*. Downers Grove, IL: InterVarsity Press, 2015.

In the context of a continuing culture war concerning homosexuality, Debra Hirsch relocates the conversation from an "us versus them" or an in-or-out orientation to a more inclusive discussion of sexuality and gender for parents and church leaders alike. Her winsome storytelling and ability to connect the lived experiences of real people with God's creative goodness in the world make this a great resource for all seeking to understand, experience and extend God's grace in the midst of conflicting messages about sexuality.

Lee, Justin. *Torn: Rescuing the Gospel from the Gays-vs.-Christians Debate*. New York: Jericho Books, 2013.

Justin Lee leads the Gay Christian Network and offers resources to gay Christians and their parents. This book offers a helpful overview of many issues Christians encounter when discussing homosexuality.

Yarhouse, Mark A. *Homosexuality and the Christian: A Guide for Parents, Pastors, and Friends*. Bloomington, MN: Bethany House, 2010.

Yarhouse offers a compassionate and thoughtful guide for parents who have questions about homosexuality and how to respond to family members who come out as gay.

Appendix B

Sexual Abuse and Violence Against Women

*L*ove is not abuse. Helping our girls understand the difference is important. Most abusers will try to convince them otherwise. This appendix contains some definitions, advice and resources to help you when talking with your girls about this difficult topic. According to the United States Department of Justice, domestic violence includes:

- physical abuse
- emotional abuse
- economic abuse
- psychological abuse
- sexual abuse[1]

The Department of Justice also defines sexual assault as "any type of sexual contact or behavior that occurs without the explicit consent of the recipient. Falling under the definition of sexual assault are such sexual activities as forced sexual intercourse, forcible sodomy, child molestation, incest, fondling, and attempted rape."[2]

The Centers for Disease Control and Prevention defines sexual violence as "any sexual act that is perpetrated against someone's will." This includes a completed nonconsensual sex act (rape), an attempted nonconsensual sex act, abusive sexual contact (such as unwanted touching) and noncontact sexual abuse (such as threatened sexual violence, exhibitionism or verbal sexual harassment). "All types involve victims who do not consent, or who are unable to consent or refuse to allow the act." The CDC offers these additional definitions:

- **Completed sex act:** contact between the penis and the vulva or the penis and the anus involving penetration, however slight; contact between the mouth and penis, vulva or anus; or penetration of the anal or genital opening of another person by a hand, finger or other object.

- **Attempted (but not completed) sex act:** an attempt at any of the above.

- **Abusive sexual contact:** intentional touching, either directly or through the clothing, of the genitalia, anus, groin, breast, inner thigh or buttocks of any person without his or her consent, or of a person who is unable to consent or refuse.

- **Noncontact sexual abuse:** abuse that does not involve physical contact of a sexual nature between perpetrator and victim. It includes voyeurism, intentional exposure of an individual to exhibitionism, unwanted exposure to pornography, verbal or behavioral sexual harassment, threats of sexual violence to accomplish some other end, or taking nude photographs of a sexual nature of another person without his or her consent or knowledge, or of a person who is unable to consent or refuse.[3]

While physical and emotional abuse are serious concerns as well, this appendix focuses on sexual abuse. The resources listed at the end include more information on dating violence and emotional abuse.

Warning Signs

Here are some signs and signals of sexual abuse, adapted from *Teaching Your Children Healthy Sexuality*:[4]

- Bed-wetting
- Sleep disturbances and nightmares
- Lack of appetite
- Fear of being left alone or with someone they have been alone with
- Depression
- Sexually acting out or sex play with dolls or toys
- Drawing naked pictures
- Acts of sexual aggression
- Learning problems in school
- Poor peer relationships
- Self-destructive behavior, cutting, taking unusual risks
- Suicidality, medicating of pain with drug and alcohol abuse
- Nervousness, aggression, disruptiveness, destructive behavior, hurting others (perhaps acting out their hurt to secure attention)
- Running away
- Seductive or promiscuous behavior
- Shutting down sexually and emotionally

- Lack of trust and hostility toward authority figures
- Fear of going home or of being left alone with the abuser
- Severe depression
- Pain, itching, bleeding, bruises in the genital area
- Extremely low self-esteem

Many survivors of sexual abuse go on to live healthy and productive lives. Some are even inspired to become advocates for victims or activists in the cause to stop sexual abuse and gender-based violence.

If it's happened to you, get help. Go to counseling, talk with a supportive friend or family member, or join an abuse recovery group. Find places and people of healing and get healed. If you don't do it for your own sake, do it for the sake of your daughter. Don't suffer in silence and don't think you are alone. Don't minimize the experience or blame yourself. Abuse is never the victim's fault.

Sexual abuse victims experience different levels of trauma depending on their circumstances, but all are traumatized to one degree or another. If we don't get help, we may fall into the trap of reenacting our trauma in our own family systems in ways that we think are normal.[5]

If it happens to your daughter, talk about it. Then talk about it again. Don't stay silent about the trauma or how it has affected your family. Don't keep it a secret. Secrecy and silence increase feelings of shame. Get help for yourself and your daughter, then keep getting help at different stages of development. Trauma gets buried and resurfaces in unexpected ways and at surprising times, so find a trusted professional to check in with regularly. Talk about it periodically as a family.

Ask your professional guide to help you talk honestly and in age-appropriate ways about your feelings and outrage at what has happened.

Don't be afraid to let your daughter see your anger and rage over the situation. It's more harmful for her to think your silence means you don't care or you're too ashamed of her to talk about it when the exact opposite is true. Learn to recognize your triggers, and when your anger leaks out, don't be afraid of it and don't stuff it. Some parents unintentionally distance themselves because they don't want their daughter to see their own hurt. Offer to embrace your daughter's pain with her and pray with her for healing, but don't force your daughter to embrace you, or the pain, or the prayers.

Healing takes time and work. One abuse victim I interviewed wished her parents had talked to her more about the abuse while she was growing up. When I asked her parents about it, her mom confessed that she couldn't talk about it for years because it made her so angry.

Much of this advice applies to victims of domestic violence as well. Domestic violence and dating violence are important topics to discuss with your daughters. Whether it's sexual abuse or dating violence, love is not abuse. And it's never the victim's fault.

Abuse affects the whole family, not just the person experiencing the abuse. But God has given us to each other to be agents of healing in one another's lives. We are called to be cooperative friends of Jesus, living lives of creative goodness in the power of the Holy Spirit for the sake of others. Together as families—along with our communities and with the help of trained mental health professionals—we *can* find healing.

Jesus revealed himself and proclaimed his mission saying:

"The Spirit of the Lord is on me,
>   because he has anointed me to preach good news to
>   the poor.

He has sent me to heal the broken hearted,
>   to proclaim release to the captives,
>   recovering of sight to the blind,
>   to deliver those who are crushed,
>   and to proclaim the acceptable year of the Lord."
>   (Luke 4:18-19, WEB)

God desires to heal, deliver, release and restore all of us. The acceptable year of the Lord has come in Jesus Christ who loves and accepts us just as we are—broken, abused, captive to fear—he takes us into his embrace and changes us forever.

Resources on Sexual Abuse and Trauma

Allender, Dan. *The Wounded Heart: Hope for Adult Victims of Childhood Sexual Abuse.* Colorado Springs, CO: NavPress, 2008.

This is an updated version of the book my sister went through as a young adult. It has been revised and updated over the years and is a standard in many Christian counseling practices for helping young adults deal with past abuse. Dan Allender continues to work with victims of abuse and offers workshops for lay counselors, professionals and those desiring personal growth. For more information on his latest resources and workshops visit theallendercenter.org.

breakthecycle.org

faithtrustinstitute.org

Kearney, Dr. R. Timothy. *Caring for Sexually Abused Children: A Handbook for Families and Churches.* Downers Grove, IL: InterVarsity Press, 2001.

This book is a great resource for families with children who have experienced sexual abuse, but it should never take the place of professional counseling. Parents often feel powerless when discovering their child has been abused, but this book is an empowering resource to help you care for your family in the midst of the trauma.

There are many online resources offering free booklets to parents and educators. Check with your local school nurse or counseling office, hospitals and medical centers for more resources.

Appendix C

Talking Topics

*Y*ou don't need to talk about every topic on this list. Some may not even seem explicitly related to sex but may be relevant to your situation. Others may not be relevant to you and your daughter at all. You may want to talk about other topics that aren't covered in this book. I encourage you to seek out a variety of resources to inform and equip you in this important parenting task.

Abortion
Abusive relationships—dating and friends
Appropriate touch and inappropriate touch
Attraction, chemistry
Beauty
Birth control
Body image
Bonding
Boundaries
Christians dating non-Christians
Clothing and modesty issues

Commitments
Consequences of sexual activity
Cross-gender friendships
Cultural influences
Date rape
Dating
Depression and sex
Developing a theology of healthy sexuality
Drug and alcohol use and abuse
Eating disorders
Emotions
Family systems and family values
Flirting
Gender differences—real and imagined
Gender identity confusion and homosexuality
Grace and forgiveness
HIV/AIDS
Hooking up/friends with benefits
Hormones
How far is too far?
Individuation
Integrity—true self, true love and so on
Internet and social media influence
Intersexuality
Intimacy
Lust
Marriage
Masturbation
Motherhood
Movie, music and other media influences
Nutrition

Oral sex

Partying

Peer pressure

PMS

Pornography

Power of friendship

Pregnancy and birth

Radical respect for the opposite sex and for others who
     are different

Romantic ideals

Secondary virginity

Self-control and self-discipline

Self-image

Setting standards

Sex's spiritual and emotional aspects (it's not just
     physical, like a sport or a game)

Sexual abuse

Sexual fantasy and imagination

Sexual intercourse

Sexual metaphors

Sexual purity pledges

Sexually transmitted diseases (STDs)

Stereotypes

Technical virginity

Temptation

Trust

Unconditional love

Unwed pregnancy

What does it mean to be human?

Why wait?

Notes

Chapter 1: Learning to Talk

[1]There are many anonymous social media sites parents should be aware of. For more information on these sites, I recommend Mark Oestreicher and Adam McLane, *A Parent's Guide to Understanding Social Media: Helping Your Teenager Navigate Life Online* (Loveland, CO: Simply Youth Ministry, 2012).

[2]Todd Hunter, *Christianity Beyond Belief: Following Jesus for the Sake of Others* (Downers Grove, IL: InterVarsity Press, 2009).

[3]Two good introductory books to begin reading on boundaries are Henry Cloud and John Townsend, *Boundaries: When to Say Yes, How to Say No to Take Control of Your Life* (Grand Rapids: Zondervan, 1992) and Melody Beattie, *The New Codependency: Help and Guidance for Today's Generation* (New York: Simon and Schuster, 2010). Henry Cloud has produced many specific follow-up books such as *Boundaries with Teens*.

[4]If you see yourself in this description, you may consider professional counseling.

[5]For a review of research on adolescent sexual behavior see Melanie J. Zimmer-Gembeck and Mark Helfand, "Ten years of longitudinal research on U.S. adolescent sexual behavior: Developmental correlates of sexual intercourse, and the importance of age, gender and ethnic background," *Developmental Review* 28, no. 2 (2008): 153-224, http://dx.doi.org/10.1016/j.dr.2007.06.001.

Chapter 2: The How-To Sex Talk

[1]Debra Haffner, *From Diapers to Dating: A Parent's Guide to Raising Sexually Healthy Children*, 2nd ed. (New York: Newmarket Press, 2008).

[2]Jane Graver and Len Ebert, *How You Are Changing: For Girls Ages 10-12 and Parents*, Learning About Sex for the Christian Family (St. Louis: Concordia Publishing House, 2008).

[3]Foster Cline and Jim Fay, *Parenting with Love and Logic: Teaching Children Responsibility* (Colorado Springs, CO: NavPress, 2006).

Chapter 3: Talking Topics: Ages Nine to Twelve

[1]Caroline Knorr, "Too Sexy, Too Soon," Common Sense Media (blog), February 8, 2011, www.commonsensemedia.org/blog/too-sexy-too-soon.

[2]Diane E. Levin and Jean Kilbourne, *So Sexy So Soon: The New Sexualized Childhood and What Parents Can Do to Protect Their Kids* (New York: Ballantine Books, 2009), p. 5.

[3]If you want to learn more, visit the Media Education Foundation website, mediaed.org, and search for *Dreamworlds 3*. On this website you will also find other educational videos about media, culture and society. The resources are designed for the classroom, but you may also be able to find shortened versions of some of the documentaries on YouTube.

[4]Emily Maynard, "The Modesty Rules: Is a Woman Responsible for a Man's Lust?" ChurchLeaders, www.churchleaders.com/pastors/pastor-articles/164005-emily-maynard-modesty-rules-is-a-woman-responsible-lust.html.

[5]Sharon Hodde Miller, "How 'Modest Is Hottest' Is Hurting Christian Women," *Her.meneutics*, Christianity Today, December 2011, www.christianitytoday.com/women/2011/december/how-modest-is-hottest-is-hurting-christian-women.html.

[6]"Child Sexual Abuse Statistics," National Center for Victims of Crime, www.victimsofcrime.org/media/reporting-on-child-sexual-abuse/child-sexual-abuse-statistics.

[7]René Girard, *Violence and the Sacred* (New York: Bloomsbury Academic, 2013), pp. 152–78.

[8]Margaret Wheatley, *Leadership and the New Science: Discovering Order in a Chaotic World* (San Francisco: Berrett-Koehler, 2006), p. 117.

Chapter 4: Where Did My Little Girl Go?

[1]"The Rose: Sexual Purity," Openers, The Source for Youth Ministry, www.thesource4ym.com/outreach/topic.aspx?ID=138.

[2]Samantha Field, "Roses: How the Purity Culture Taught Me to Be Abused," Defeating the Dragons (blog), January 31, 2013, defeatingthedragons.wordpress.com/2013/01/31/51/; Sarah Galo, "How Not to Talk About Purity," *Relevant Magazine*, April 28, 2014, www.relevantmagazine.com/god/church/how-not-talk-about-purity.

[3]Lisa Graham McMinn, *Sexuality and Holy Longing: Embracing Intimacy in a Broken World* (San Francisco: Jossey-Bass, 2004), p.16.

[4]Ibid., p. 20.

Chapter 6: The How-Not-To Sex Talk

[1]"(Almost) Everyone's Doing It," *Relevant Magazine* 53 (September/October 2011): 65, www.relevantmagazine.com/life/relationships/almost-everyones-doing-it.

[2]John Blake, "Why young christians aren't waiting anymore," CNN Belief Blog, September 27, 2011, religion.blogs.cnn.com/2011/09/27/why-young-christians-arent-waiting-anymore.

[3]Jessica Valenti, *The Purity Myth: How America's Obsession with Virginity Is Hurting Young Women* (Berkeley, CA: Seal Press, 2009), p. 9.

[4]For more detailed information on the harmful potential of purity pledges see Jessica Valenti, *The Purity Myth: How America's Obsession with Virginity is Hurting Young Women* (Berkeley, CA: Seal Press, 2009) and Dianna Anderson, *Damaged Goods: New Perspectives on Christian Purity* (New York: Jericho Books, 2015).

[5]Bibledex: A Video About Every Book in the Bible, University of Nottingham, www.bibledex.com.

[6]David Kinnaman, *You Lost Me: Why Young Christians Are Leaving the Church* (Grand Rapids: Baker Books, 2011), p. 23.

Chapter 7: Talking Topics: Ages Thirteen to Seventeen

[1]John and Julie Gottman, *The Seven Principles for Making Marriage Work: A Practical Guide from the Country's Foremost Relationship Expert* (New York: Crown Publishers, 1999).

Chapter 8: Fear Factor

[1]Rob Bell, *Sex God: Exploring the Endless Connections between Sexuality and Spirituality* (Grand Rapids: Zondervan, 2007), p. 136.

[2]See Brené Brown, "Listening to Shame," TED Talk, March 2012, www.ted.com/talks/brene_brown_listening_to_shame.

Chapter 9: Overcoming Fear and Shame

[1]Visit www.thankgodforsex.org for more information and to join a community solidarity for those who've experienced religious sexual shame.

[2]Catherine Skurja with Jen Johnson, *Paradox Lost: Uncovering Your True*

Identity in Christ (North Plains, OR: Imago Dei Ministries, 2012).

Appendix B: Sexual Abuse and Violence Against Women

[1]"What Is Domestic Violence?" US Department of Justice, July 23, 2014, www.ovw.usdoj.gov/domviolence.htm.

[2]"What Is Sexual Assault?" US Department of Justice, July 23, 2014, www.ovw.usdoj.gov/sexassault.htm.

[3]"Sexual Violence: Definitions," Centers for Disease Control and Prevention, www.cdc.gov/violenceprevention/sexualviolence/definitions.html.

[4]Adapted from Jim Burns, *Teaching Your Children Healthy Sexuality: A Biblical Approach to Prepare Them for Life*, Pure Foundations for Parents (Bloomington, MN: Bethany House, 2008).

[5]Serene Jones, *Trauma and Grace: Theology in a Ruptured World* (Louisville, KY: Westminster John Knox, 2009), p. 65.

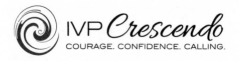
COURAGE. CONFIDENCE. CALLING.

Some voices challenge us. Others support or encourage us. Voices can move us to change our minds, draw close to God, discover a new spiritual gift. The voices of others are shaping who we are.

The voices behind IVP Crescendo join together to draw us into God's story. We'll discover God's work around the globe even as we learn to love the people around the corner. We'll have opportunity to heal our places of pain. We'll discover new ways to love our families. We'll hear God's voice speaking into our lives as we discover new places of influence.

IVP Crescendo invites you to join in the rising chorus

- *to listen to the voices of others*
- *to hear the voice of God*
- *and to grow your own voice in*

COURAGE. CONFIDENCE. CALLING.

ivpress.com/crescendo
ivpress.com/crescendo-social